T0198214

Advances in Technology for the Sleep Field

Editor

STEVEN J. HOLFINGER

SLEEP MEDICINE CLINICS

www.sleep.theclinics.com

September 2023 • Volume 18 • Number 3

ELSEVIER

1600 John F. Kennedy Boulevard • Suite 1800 • Philadelphia, Pennsylvania, 19103-2899

http://www.theclinics.com

SLEEP MEDICINE CLINICS Volume 18, Number 3
September 2023, ISSN 1556-407X, ISBN-13: 978-0-443-18240-2

Editor: Joanna Gascoine
Developmental Editor: Axell Ivan Jade M. Purificacion

Sleep Medicine Clinics (ISSN 1556-407X) is published quarterly by Elsevier Inc., 360 Park Avenue South, New York, NY 10010-1710. Months of issue are March, June, September and December. Business and Editorial Offices: 1600 John F. Kennedy Blvd., Ste. 1800, Philadelphia, PA 19103-2899. Customer Service Office: 3251 Riverport Lane, Maryland Heights, MO 63043. Periodicals postage paid at New York, NY and additional mailing offices. Subscription prices are $243.00 per year (US individuals), $100.00 (US and Canadian students), $612.00 (US institutions), $283.00 (Canadian individuals), $278.00 (international individuals) $135.00 (International students), $692.00 (Canadian and International institutions). Foreign air speed delivery is included in all *Clinics* subscription prices. All prices are subject to change without notice. **POSTMASTER:** Send change of address to *Sleep Medicine Clinics*, Elsevier Health Sciences Division, Subscription Customer Service, 3251 Riverport Lane, Maryland Heights, MO 63043. Customer Service: **Tel: 1-800-654-2452 (U.S. and Canada); 314-447-8871 (outside U.S. and Canada). Fax: 314-447-8029. E-mail: journalscustomerservice-usa@elsevier.com (for print support); journalsonline-support-usa@elsevier.com (for online support).**

Reprints. For copies of 100 or more of articles in this publication, please contact the Commercial Reprints Department, Elsevier Inc., 360 Park Avenue South, New York, NY 10010-1710. Tel.: 212-633-3874; Fax: 212-633-3820; E-mail: reprints@elsevier.com.

Sleep Medicine Clinics is covered in *MEDLINE/PubMed (Index Medicus)*.

SLEEP MEDICINE CLINICS

FORTHCOMING ISSUES

December 2023
Sleep in Women
Monica Andersen, *Editor*

March 2024
The Parasomnias
Alon Y. Avidan, *Editor*

RECENT ISSUES

June 2023
Pediatric Sleep Clinics
Haviva Veler, *Editor*

March 2023
Adjunct Interventions to Cognitive Behavioral Therapy for Insomnia
Joshua Hyong-Jin-Cho, *Editor*

SERIES OF RELATED INTEREST

Neurologic Clinics
https://www.neurologic.theclinics.com/

THE CLINICS ARE AVAILABLE ONLINE!
Access your subscription at:
www.theclinics.com

Contributors

CONSULTING EDITORS

TEOFILO LEE-CHIONG Jr, MD
Professor of Medicine, National Jewish Health,
Professor of Medicine, University of Colorado,
Denver, Colorado, USA; Chief Medical Liaison,
Philips Respironics, Murrysville, Pennsylvania,
USA

ANA C. KRIEGER, MD, MPH, FCCP, FAASM
Chief, Division of Sleep Neurology, Medical
Director, Weill Cornell Center for Sleep
Medicine, Professor of Clinical Medicine,
Professor of Medicine in Neurology and Genetic
Medicine, Weill Cornell Medical College,
Cornell University, New York, New York, USA

EDITOR

STEVEN J. HOLFINGER, MD, MS
Assistant Clinical Professor, Associate Sleep
Fellowship Director, Department of Internal

Medicine, Division of Pulmonary, Critical Care
and Sleep Medicine, The Ohio State University,
Columbus, Ohio, USA

AUTHORS

DIEGO ALVAREZ-ESTEVEZ, PhD
Center for Information and Communications
Technology Research (CITIC), Universidade da
Coruña, Spain

SÉBASTIEN BAILLIEUL, MD, PhD
Univ. Grenoble Alpes, HP2 (Hypoxia and Physio-
Pathologies) Laboratory, Inserm (French National
Institute of Health and Medical Research) U1300,
Sleep Laboratory, Grenoble Alpes University
Hospital Center, Grenoble, France

SÉBASTIEN BAILLY, PharmD, PhD
Univ. Grenoble Alpes, HP2 (Hypoxia and
Physio-Pathologies) Laboratory, Inserm
(French National Institute of Health and
Medical Research) U1300, Sleep Laboratory,
Grenoble Alpes University Hospital Center,
Grenoble, France

KATHLEEN R. BILLINGS, MD
Division of Pediatric Otolaryngology–Head
and Neck Surgery, Ann & Robert H. Lurie
Children's Hospital of Chicago, Department
of Otolaryngology–Head and Neck
Surgery, Northwestern University Feinberg
School of Medicine, Chicago, Illinois,
USA

JUDITE BLANC, PhD
Department of Psychiatry and Behavioral
Sciences, University of Miami Miller School of
Medicine, Center for Translational Sleep and
Circadian Sciences (TSCS), Miami, Florida,
USA

MATTHEW BOHN, BS
Behavioral Biology Branch, Walter Reed Army
Institute of Research, Silver Spring, Maryland,
USA

MARY CARRASCO, BS
Department of Psychiatry and Behavioral
Sciences, University of Miami Miller
School of Medicine, Department of Informatics
and Health Data Science, The Media
and Innovation Lab, Miami, Florida,
USA

AMBROSE A. CHIANG, MD, FCCP, FAASM
Division of Sleep Medicine, Louis Stokes
Cleveland VA Medical Center, Division of
Pulmonary, Critical Care, and Sleep Medicine,
University Hospitals Cleveland Medical Center,
Department of Medicine, Case Western
Reserve University, Cleveland, Ohio,
USA

JACOB COLLEN, MD
Department of Medicine, Uniformed Services University of the Health Sciences, Pulmonary, Critical Care and Sleep Medicine, Walter Reed National Military Medical Center, Bethesda, Maryland, USA

SEAN DEERING, BS
Sleep, Tactical Efficiency and Endurance Lab, Warfighter Performance Department, Naval Health Research Center, Leidos, Inc, San Diego, California, USA

TRACY JILL DOTY, PhD
Behavioral Biology Branch, Walter Reed Army Institute of Research, Silver Spring, Maryland, USA

LUNTHITA M. DUTHELY, EdD
Obstetrics, Gynecology and Reproductive Sciences, Department of Public Health Sciences, University of Miami Miller School of Medicine, Don Soffer Clinical Research Center

ALISON FOOTE, PhD
Sleep Laboratory, Grenoble Alpes University Hospital Center, Grenoble, France

LAURA FRANCOIS, BS
Department of Psychiatry and Behavioral Sciences, University of Miami Miller School of Medicine

ANNE GERMAIN, PhD
NOCTEM Health Inc, Pittsburgh, Pennsylvania, USA

INDIRA GURUBHAGAVATULA, MD
Division of Sleep Medicine, Perelman School of Medicine, University of Pennsylvania, Corporal Michael J. Crescenz Deparment of Veterans Affairs Medical Center, Philadelphia, Pennsylvania, USA

KAITLYN HAHN, BS
Department of Psychiatry and Behavioral Sciences, University of Miami Miller School of Medicine, Miami, Florida, USA

CAMILLA M. HOYOS, MPH, PhD
Centre for Sleep and Chronobiology, Woolcock Institute of Medical Research, The University of Sydney, Faculty of Science, School of Psychology and Brain and Mind Centre, Sydney, Australia

GIRARDIN JEAN-LOUIS, PhD
Department of Psychiatry and Behavioral Sciences, University of Miami Miller School of Medicine, CRB, Translational Sleep and Circadian Sciences (TSCS), Miami, Florida, USA

TYLER JOHNSON, MD
Division of Sleep Medicine, Perelman School of Medicine, University of Pennsylvania, Philadelphia, Pennsylvania, USA

SEEMA KHOSLA, MD, FCCP, FAASM
North Dakota Center for Sleep, Fargo, North Dakota, USA

ROO KILLICK, MBBS, FRACP, PhD
Centre for Sleep and Chronobiology, Woolcock Institute of Medical Research, The University of Sydney, Sydney, Australia

GRACE KLOSTERMAN, BS
Behavioral Biology Branch, Walter Reed Army Institute of Research, Silver Spring, Maryland, USA

ANDREW G. KUBALA, PhD
Sleep, Tactical Efficiency and Endurance Lab, Warfighter Performance Department, Naval Health Research Center, Leidos, Inc, San Diego, California, USA

ALICE D. LAGOY, PhD
Sleep, Tactical Efficiency and Endurance Lab, Warfighter Performance Department, Naval Health Research Center, Leidos, Inc, San Diego, California, USA

JOHN MADDALOZZO, MD
Division of Pediatric Otolaryngology–Head and Neck Surgery, Ann & Robert H. Lurie Children's Hospital of Chicago, Department of Otolaryngology–Head and Neck Surgery, Northwestern University Feinberg School of Medicine, Chicago, Illinois, USA

RACHEL R. MARKWALD, PhD
Sleep, Tactical Efficiency and Endurance Lab, Warfighter Performance Department, Naval Health Research Center, San Diego, California, USA

JEAN-BENOÎT MARTINOT, MD
Sleep Laboratory, CHU Université Catholique de Louvain (UCL) Namur Site Sainte-Elisabeth, Namur, Belgium; Institute of Experimental and Clinical Research, UCL Bruxelles Woluwe, Brussels, Belgium

RAOUA BEN MESSAOUD, PhD
Univ. Grenoble Alpes, HP2 (Hypoxia and Physio-Pathologies) Laboratory, Inserm (French National Institute of Health and Medical Research) U1300, Sleep Laboratory, Grenoble Alpes University Hospital Center, Grenoble, France

JESSE MOORE, MS
Department of Psychiatry and Behavioral Sciences, University of Miami Miller School of Medicine, Department of Informatics and Health Data Science, The Media and Innovation Lab, Miami, Florida, USA

BRUNO OLIVEIRA, BS
Department of Psychiatry and Behavioral Sciences, University of Miami Miller School of Medicine, Miami, Florida, USA

ALLAN I. PACK, MBChB, PhD
John Miclot Professor of Medicine, Division of Sleep Medicine, Department of Medicine, University of Pennsylvania, Perelman School of Medicine, Philadelphia, Pennsylvania, USA

JEAN-LOUIS PÉPIN, MD, PhD
Univ. Grenoble Alpes, HP2 (Hypoxia and Physio-Pathologies) Laboratory, Inserm (French National Institute of Health and Medical Research) U1300, Sleep Laboratory, Grenoble Alpes University Hospital Center, Grenoble, France

RO'MYA PHILLIPS, BS
Florida Atlantic University, Boca Raton, Florida, USA

AZIZI A. SEIXAS, PhD
Department of Psychiatry and Behavioral Sciences, University of Miami Miller School of Medicine, CRB, Translational Sleep and Circadian Sciences (TSCS), Department of Informatics and Health Data Science, The Media and Innovation Lab, Miami, Florida, USA

GUIDO SIMONELLI, MD
Behavioral Biology Branch, Walter Reed Army Institute of Research, Silver Spring, Maryland, USA; Department of Medicine and Neuroscience, Faculty of Medicine, Université de Montréal, Centre d'études avancées en médecine du sommeil, Hôpital du Sacré-Coeur de Montréal, Montréal, Québec, Canada

EMILY K. STEKL, BA
Behavioral Biology Branch, Walter Reed Army Institute of Research, Silver Spring, Maryland, USA

CANDICE A. STERNBERG, MD
Department of Infectious Diseases, University of Miami Miller School of Medicine, Miami, Florida, USA

LACHLAN STRANKS, MBBS
Centre for Sleep and Chronobiology, Woolcock Institute of Medical Research, The University of Sydney, Sydney, Australia; The University of Adelaide, Faculty of Health and Medical Sciences, Adelaide, Australia

RENAUD TAMISIER, MD, PhD
Univ. Grenoble Alpes, HP2 (Hypoxia and Physio-Pathologies) Laboratory, Inserm (French National Institute of Health and Medical Research) U1300, Sleep Laboratory, Grenoble Alpes University Hospital Center, Grenoble, France

Contents

challenging. An approach to ascertain them using a simple model of ventilatory control has been proposed. It is based, however, on untenable assumptions. There are limited validation data and reproducibility is not stellar. There are also different symptom subtypes. They have been found in multiple population-based and clinical cohorts worldwide. Symptomatic benefit from therapy is most marked in the excessively sleepy subtype. This group may also be the group at increased CV risk from obstructive sleep apnea.

Sleep apnea is nowadays recognized as a treatable chronic disease and awareness of it has increased, leading to an upsurge in demand for diagnostic testing. Conventionally, diagnosis depends on overnight polysomnography in a sleep clinic, which is highly human-resource intensive and ignores the night-to-night variability in classical sleep apnea markers, such as the apnea–hypopnea index. In this review, the authors summarize the main improvements that could be made in the sleep apnea diagnosis strategy; how technological innovations and multi-night home testing could be used to simplify, increase access, and reduce costs of diagnostic testing while avoiding misclassification of severity.

As the importance of good sleep continues to gain public recognition, the market for sleep-monitoring devices continues to grow. Modern technology has shifted from simple sleep tracking to a more granular sleep health assessment. We examine the available functionalities of consumer wearable sleep trackers (CWSTs) and how they perform in healthy individuals and disease states. Additionally, the continuum of sleep technology from consumer-grade to medical-grade is detailed. As this trend invariably grows, we urge professional societies to develop guidelines encompassing the practical clinical use of CWSTs and how best to incorporate them into patient care plans.

Epidemiologic studies have demonstrated that short sleep duration is associated with an increased risk of cardio-metabolic health outcomes including cardiovascular disease mortality, coronary heart disease, type 2 diabetes mellitus, hypertension, and metabolic syndrome. Experimental sleep restriction studies have sought to explain these findings. This review describes the main evidence of these associations and possible mechanisms explaining them. Whether sleep extension reverses these now widely acknowledged adverse health effects and the feasibility of implementing such strategies on a public health level is discussed.

This article summarizes the definitions of vigilance, fatigue, and sleepiness, as well as tools used in their assessment. Consideration is given to the strengths and limitations of the different subjective and objective tools. Future directions for research are also discussed, as well as the public health importance of continued investigation in this subject.

Dawn of a New Dawn: Advances in Sleep Health to Optimize Performance 361

Alice D. LaGoy, Andrew G. Kubala, Sean Deering, Anne Germain, and Rachel R. Markwald

Optimal sleep health is a critical component to high-level performance. In populations such as the military, public service (eg, firefighters), and health care, achieving optimal sleep health is difficult and subsequently deficiencies in sleep health may lead to performance decrements. However, advances in sleep monitoring technologies and mitigation strategies for poor sleep health show promise for further ecological scientific investigation within these populations. The current review briefly outlines the relationship between sleep health and performance as well as current advances in behavioral and technological approaches to improving sleep health for performance.

A 2022 Survey of Commercially Available Smartphone Apps for Sleep: Most Enhance Sleep 373

Tracy Jill Doty, Emily K. Stekl, Matthew Bohn, Grace Klosterman, Guido Simonelli, and Jacob Collen

Commercially available smartphone apps represent an ever-evolving and fast-growing market. Our review systematically surveyed currently available commercial sleep smartphone apps to provide details to inform both providers and patients alike, in addition to the healthy consumer market. Most current sleep apps offer a free version and are designed to be used while awake, prior to sleep, and focus on the enhancement of sleep, rather than measurement, by targeting sleep latency using auditory stimuli. Sleep apps could be considered a possible strategy for patients and consumers to improve their sleep, although further validation of specific apps is recommended.

Preface
Envisioning Tomorrow Using Dawn's First Light

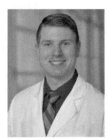

Steven J. Holfinger, MD, MS
Editor

The most certain attribute of the future is how difficult it can be to predict; however, the developing tidal wave of technology within the field of sleep medicine appears to be both inevitable in its coming and incalculable in its impact.

Just over 100 years ago, it would have been difficult to envision the evolution of cardiology as the first cardiac catheterization was performed in humans. Yet in retrospect, we can see that periodic breakthroughs with rapid change occurred amid years of slow growth. While catheterization was initially used as a hemodynamic measurement tool for many decades, its bedside use was uncommon until the invention of the "Swan-Ganz" catheter in 1970. Today's primary use for the treatment of myocardial infarction was not realized until the 1980s, with this discovery leading to rapid clinical expansion to more than a million cardiac catheterizations a year in the United States alone.

Sleep technologies are similarly on the verge of breakthroughs on several key fronts. From the standpoint of clinical sleep measurement, artificial intelligence–assisted scoring is nearly ready for widespread clinical use. How artificial intelligence should be used, and perhaps more importantly, its limitations, will be imperative to using it correctly and equitably.

The impact of consumer devices on clinical decision making may be the most difficult change to forecast. Sleep tracking has become ubiquitous among wearable devices with the capacity to do so, yet the performance of these devices remains questionable in the clinical realm. Nevertheless, when reputable companies produce a device, the public perception of accuracy drives sales more than data-driven metrics. As consumer devices continue to blur the line between recreational use and their clinical counterparts, more and more patients will seek expertise based on reports from their sleep-tracking devices. While it may seem daunting for clinicians to understand the variety of apps and devices available to the public, the technology will reach a point where clinicians will be expected to interpret the results. Instead of resisting change, sleep medicine experts will need to learn how to best utilize this new information. These consumer devices may open the door to longitudinal monitoring, generate methods to analyze the sleep environment, or create metrics to better quantify vague symptoms like fatigue. The devices may also unlock barriers to previously unreachable populations, for instance, in patients who underestimate their own self-harm, as is the case for patients with insufficient sleep syndrome. In addition, these devices may also reach

Sleep Med Clin 18 (2023) xiii–xiv
https://doi.org/10.1016/j.jsmc.2023.06.001
1556-407X/23/© 2023 Published by Elsevier Inc.

underserved, oppressed, and/or marginalized communities with less access and trust in professional health care.

Sleep-disordered breathing remains at the forefront of clinical encounters, and conventional therapies are unable to treat every scenario. Combining traditional and integrative medicine approaches can give insight into how we can shift our standard treatment approach to utilize the available options.

As we look forward, the most exciting aspects of sleep medicine are likely yet to be discovered. How rapidly and effectively we can translate these new technologies into clinical applications will make a tremendous impact on our patients' lives.

Steven J. Holfinger, MD, MS
Department of Internal Medicine
Division of Pulmonary, Critical Care & Sleep
Medicine
The Ohio State University
2012 Kenny Road #215
Columbus, OH, 43221, USA

E-mail address:
Steven.Holfinger@osumc.edu

Bringing Health Care Equity to Diverse and Underserved Populations in Sleep Medicine and Research Through a Digital Health Equity Framework

Judite Blanc, PhD[a], Kaitlyn Hahn, BS[b], Bruno Oliveira, BS[c],
Ro'Mya Phillips, BS[d], Lunthita M. Duthely, EdD[e], Laura Francois, BS[b],
Mary Carrasco, BS[b,f], Jesse Moore, MS[b,f], Candice A. Sternberg, MD[g],
Girardin Jean-Louis, PhD[h], Azizi A. Seixas, PhD[a,b,f,*]

KEYWORDS

- Sleep health • Equity • Digital health • Population health

KEY POINTS

- By collecting and analyzing data on sleep health outcomes, health care providers can identify disparities in sleep quality, duration, and disorders. This can lead to targeted interventions that improve sleep health equity.
- Improving access to care, promoting patient engagement and empowerment, providing personalized care, coordinating care, and using data-driven decision making can all contribute to promoting sleep health equity.
- Addressing the unique cultural, social, and economic factors that affect a patient's sleep health can help reduce disparities in sleep health outcomes.

INTRODUCTION

The declaration of the novel coronavirus disease 2019 (COVID-19) pandemic in 2020 disrupted biomedical research and clinical care practices in medicine, most notably in sleep medicine and research.[1] Minoritized communities (racial, ethnic minorities, and low-income individuals) were

[a] Department of Psychiatry and Behavioral Sciences, University of Miami Miller School of Medicine, Center for Translational Sleep and Circadian Sciences (TSCS), Clinical Research Building, 14th Floor 1120 Northwest 14th Street, Room 1448, Miami, FL 33136, USA; [b] Department of Psychiatry and Behavioral Sciences, University of Miami Miller School of Medicine; [c] Department of Psychiatry and Behavioral Sciences, University of Miami Miller School of Medicine, 1120 Northwest 14th Street, 14th Floor, Suite 1451A, Miami, FL 33136, USA; [d] Florida Atlantic University, 777 Glades Road, Boca Raton, FL 33431, USA; [e] Obstetrics, Gynecology & Reproductive Sciences, Department of Public Health Sciences, University of Miami Miller School of Medicine, Don Soffer Clinical Research Center 1162; [f] Department of Informatics and Health Data Science, The Media and Innovation Lab, 1120 Northwest 14th Street, Room 1452, Miami, FL 33136, USA; [g] Department of Infectious Diseases, University of Miami Miller School of Medicine, Clinical Research Building, 1120 Northwest 14th Street #858, Miami, FL 33136, USA; [h] Department of Psychiatry and Behavioral Sciences, University of Miami Miller School of Medicine, CRB, Translational Sleep and Circadian Sciences (TSCS), 14th Floor 1120 Northwest 14th Street, Room 1449, Miami, FL 33136, USA

* Corresponding author. University of Miami Miller School of Medicine, 1120 NW 14th Street Miami, FL 33136.
E-mail address: azizi.seixas@med.miami.edu

Sleep Med Clin 18 (2023) 255–267
https://doi.org/10.1016/j.jsmc.2023.05.009
1556-407X/23/© 2023 Elsevier Inc. All rights reserved.

disproportionately affected by COVID-19, with high infection, hospitalizations, and mortality rates and restricted access to health services.[2] These poor health outcomes are partly caused by the high rate of medical comorbidities and increased mistrust toward medical professionals.[3] To overcome these health differences and disparities, it is imperative to include individuals from diverse and minoritized populations (eg, racial/ethnic and low-income groups) who are less likely to participate in biomedical research and underutilize health care services.[4] There are unique challenges associated with engaging, enrolling, and treating individuals from minoritized populations in medicine, particularly sleep research and health care. Some of these challenges are caused by deep structural and social determinants of health (eg, safe housing and neighborhoods, transportation, racism, discrimination, and violence, education, job opportunities, low income, limited access to healthy foods, polluted air and water, language barriers, and low health literacy skills).[5] Since the onset of the pandemic, digital solutions, mobile health, and telehealth solutions have proliferated to increase patients' access to research and clinical care services. However, wide-scale implementation and dissemination of these solutions, especially in minoritized populations and communities, have been hindered by the limited access to quality Internet access, low digital literacy and self-efficacy (knowing how to and feeling comfortable using digital devices), and significant mistrust in the privacy and security of technology, which the authors classify as the digital divide. To solve this digital divide in biomedical research and clinical care, the authors created a digital health equity model that identifies and solves unique intrapersonal, interpersonal, institutional, and community-based barriers that prevent access to and participation in biomedical research and clinical care.

Intrapersonal and Psychosocial Barriers

Interpersonal and psychosocial barriers, like an individual's life circumstances (social demands) and their attitudes, beliefs, and knowledge (health literacy), have prevented minoritized communities from accessing quality health care and participating in biomedical research. Structurally and administratively, biomedical research and medicine are not patient-centric, as they are time-consuming, burdensome, and inconvenient for participants and patients. For example, long and inconvenient commutes to clinical and research settings, inflexible and restrictive appointment scheduling and operational hours, and rigid eligibility research criteria systematically disqualify minoritized

communities from participating in research or clinical care (eg, sleep medicine).[6] Attitudes, beliefs, and knowledge (health literacy) are another category of intrapersonal barriers that negatively affect participation in biomedical research and clinical care. For many individuals from minoritized communities, low literacy about the importance of sleep health, the inability to identify sleep disturbances and understand their potentially adverse effects on overall health and well-being, and low health-seeking behaviors for sleep problems can lead to severe and seemingly intractable health disparities.[7] Low health literacy has been linked with unhealthy lifestyle behaviors and poor clinical outcomes.[8] Historically, individuals from minoritized and immigrant communities report lower levels of health literacy relative to majority white populations.[9,10]

Interpersonal Barriers

One significant interpersonal barrier that prevents minoritized communities from participating in biomedical research and clinical care is the implicit bias of research and health care teams. Implicit biases are unconscious and automatic associations that affect the attitudes, decisions, judgments, and behavior of research and clinical teams. In a systematic review, one-third of the 65 studies revealed that researchers' perspectives and implicit biases negatively impacted interpersonal interactions between research participants and research teams. Minoritized groups felt discouraged from participating in research studies.[5] Positive interpersonal interactions between participants and researchers are necessary for building trust through transparency and accountability. Research teams with low cultural intelligence and competence (eg, drive, action, knowledge, and strategy) are more likely to engender mistrust among patients and research participants, resulting in lower participation of minoritized individuals. Employing a digital equity model may allow teams to address implicit biases and raise cultural intelligence.[11,12]

Other interpersonal barriers include language and cultural differences, which may impede participation in biomedical research and engagement in the health care system. Language barriers negatively affect communication between medical providers and patients.[13] Individuals who experience language barriers are primarily neglected in biomedical research and health care, as research and clinical teams usually focus on recruiting anglophones. Recruitment of minoritized groups requires time and resources to learn what methods may work in certain communities to improve community acceptance of biomedical research and clinical services. To address language barriers, the authors' team ensures that all patient/participant-facing materials are culturally and linguistically tailored. This process entails translating all written and external communication materials into the target communities' preferred and accepted languages and ensuring that all engagement materials are delivered by culturally trained and competent staff. Having culturally trained and competent staff allows research and clinical teams to identify and understand barriers minoritized communities face that prevent them from participating in research and engaging with the health care system.[14] Although assessing the perceived barriers to research participation for minoritized groups is critical, it is equally important to ensure that research and clinical teams are diverse, because patients/participants in research or clinical care have less mistrust and are more willing to participate if teams are racially or culturally congruent with them. This does not mean that "skin folk makes kin folk," where having diverse representation on teams automatically earns trust by minoritized communities. Having a diverse team communicates an invaluable message of inclusivity to participants/patients, where difference is acknowledged, accepted, and welcomed. Over 2 decades of leading a health equity research program, the authors have learned that having a diverse team makes participants/patients feel safe and, thus, more motivated and willing to participate in biomedical research.

Institutional and Systemic Barriers

The third category of barriers is institutional/systemic. The long history of medical mistreatment of minoritized communities has impacted how individuals engage with research and health care.[4] To overcome deep-seated mistrust among individuals from minoritized communities, building trust between communities and biomedical and health care institutions and systems is critical.[15] A trusting environment may be promoted by encouraging high transparency between researchers, participants, providers, and patients. This is partially achieved by ensuring that potential participants/patients comprehend the entire research and clinical care journey. First, the informed consent process must be presented transparently and understandably. Participants/patients must be aware of the protections to prevent mistreatment and feel that the study staff is accessible if any questions or issues arise.[15] The authors' group implements a novel informed consent process in which a community steering committee (CSC)

cocreates the informed consent document to ensure that empowering language is embedded. For example, participants/patients are always given the flexibility to personalize their experience in biomedical research studies, as long as the fidelity of key procedures is not compromised. The authors' recruitment process is also novel, as the authors pursue a robust community engagement program, recruiting at community-based organizations, barber shops/salons, faith-based organizations, food pantries, health fairs, sporting events, and other community venues. Re-examining recruitment and participation processes has successfully increased the representation of minoritized communities in biomedical research and clinical care **Fig. 1**.

SOLUTIONS TO INCREASE PARTICIPATION OF MINORITIZED COMMUNITIES IN SLEEP RESEARCH AND MEDICINE

Despite substantial efforts to address sleep disparities and inequities, the fields of sleep research and medicine still have a far way to achieving health equity and justice for all. To achieve equity and justice in sleep research and medicine, the authors' research group in tandem with the Sleep Health Disparities Workgroup (a group of community stakeholders) has spent decades implementing community-based strategies to achieve sleep health equity.[16,17] In its sleep health equity program, the authors' group identified sleep health equity barriers and proposed policies solutions and workgroup initiatives that have the potential to advance sleep health equity (**Table 1**).

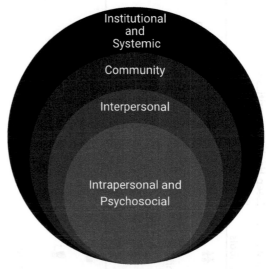

Fig. 1. Barriers in participating in sleep medicine and research.

Table 1
Ten ways the Sleep Health Disparities Working Group advanced sleep health equity

Symbols	Sleep Health Equity Barrier	Proposed Policies	Sleep Health Disparities Workgroup Initiatives
Children	1. Higher prevalence of sleep-disordered-breathing (SBD) among African–American children	Implementation of programs for sleep health literacy, early screening, and treatment for sleep disorders beginning in elementary schools Require schools at all levels to include a module on sleep health in their curriculum and referrals of at-risk youth to sleep health centers	Implementing an intervention to evaluate the effect of sleep aid and mobile applications to advance sleep health among children from low-income communities in the United States Audio-based mobile sleep aid and solutions have proven to improve sleep health in a racially diverse parent and child dyad sample[18]
Adults	2. Greater exposure to environmental risk factors for poor sleep among racial/ethnic minorities living in disadvantaged neighborhoods	Implementing a multilevel approach to reducing ecological factors that disturb sleep, such as inadequate light, noise, allergens and irritants, and air pollution. Suggestions of limitations or suppression of all sources of inadequate light, noise, allergen, irritants, and air pollution during the sleep period in identified communities	*Determinants of Insufficient Sleep Among Blacks, and Effects on Disparities in Health Outcomes (ESSENTIAL) Study* The study aims to ascertain the psychosocial (social network and psychological health) and environmental determinants (social capital, neighborhood, and built environment) of insufficient sleep *Mechanisms of Sleep Deficiency and Effects on Brain Injury and Neurocognitive Functions Among Older Blacks (MOSAIC) study* The purpose of this study was to assess the determinants of sleep deficiency and delineate their potential role in explaining observed disparities in the brain health of older Black people, indexed by novel Alzheimer disease (AD) brain biomarkers and examinations of cognitive impairment in a multicultural community sample *Determinants of Insufficient Sleep in Rural-Urban Settings (DORMIR) study* This study provides multilevel evidence supporting epidemiological findings of greater rates of insufficient sleep among Latinos/as that may explain their disproportionate burden of cardiovascular diseases (CVD) risk; the findings can lead to actionable clinical, lifestyle, and policy interventions to improve health[19]

Adults	3. A higher rate of short sleep duration increases cardiovascular risk among individuals of African descent and other minorities	Adopt a multilevel community-oriented sleep health and promotion education campaign (eg, PEERS-ED, TASHE, and MetSO) Provide incentives to corporate wellness programs that promote sleep and population health among racial/ethnic communities	*Metabolic Syndrome Outcome Study (MetSO)* The MetSO trial has shown that phone-delivered sleep education addressing impediments to OSA (obstructive sleep apnea) care among Blacks was successful in increasing OSA evaluation; the trial demonstrated that tailored OSA education is critical to increasing adherence to recommended OSA care *Tailored Approach to Sleep Health Education (TASHE)* In the TASHE trial, the authors found that Web-based sleep education significantly increased OSA self-efficacy among Blacks *PEERS-ED* This randomized controlled trial examined the role of congruent peer sleep educators and social support PEERS-ED in navigating Blacks seeking OSA care[7]
	4. Racial/ethnic minorities, particularly Blacks, are exposed to higher rates of racial discrimination, which induce stress that undermines sleep	A national campaign to raise awareness of the harmful effects of racial bias, racial profiling, and discrimination on health Increase the severity of sanctions against racial discrimination nationwide	To advance data on the impact of discrimination, the level of exposure to daily discrimination is captured through the ESSENTIAL, MOSAIC, and DORMIR community-based sleep studies investigated among Blacks and Hispanics
	5. Blacks are disproportionately concerned with the effects of particular work shifts, and need stronger work schedule regulations	Limitations of shift length, regulation of time between shifts, and regulation of the degree of circadian phase changes in consecutive workdays	Advancing research at the community level; the authors' team measured the impact of shift work and lifestyle on sufficient sleep among Blacks and Latinos This problem is captured through ESSENTIAL, MOSAIC, and DORMIR, which started before COVID The ESSENTIAL and MOSAIC projects are tailored to Blacks between the ages of 18 and 65 years old who experienced insufficient sleep, while DORMIR focuses on Hispanic/Latinos

(continued on next page)

Table 1
(continued)

Symbols	Sleep Health Equity Barrier	Proposed Policies	Sleep Health Disparities Workgroup Initiatives
Adults	6. Cultural and language barriers limit access to sleep health literacy among racial/ethnic minorities	Establishment of sleep centers with multiethnic and multilingual staff in vulnerable communities Require health care facilities in vulnerable communities to have a multiethnic and multilingual staff	The sleep health disparities workgroup evolved into a project of a multiethnic center to advance the science of sleep and circadian sciences (TSCS) in low-income communities The study PREDICT - *Precision Recruitment and Engagement of Diabetics and Hypertensives in Clinical Studies* - aimed to form/educate, engage, support, and navigate participants and providers through the process of clinical trial participation via personalization Ultimately, the authors aimed to develop solutions addressing patient, provider, and system-level barriers preventing clinical trial participation This study provides a foundation for future research to circumvent barriers preventing vulnerable communities from participating in clinical trials
	7. Poor adherence to treatment of sleep disorders among minorities, particularly Blacks at risk for OSA	A tailored behavioral intervention to increase adherence to physician recommendations (eg, MetSO and PEERS-ED studies) Requirement for cultural competency training in sleep medicine programs	In the METSO trial, the authors observed phone-delivered sleep education addressing impediments to OSA care among Blacks that successfully increased OSA evaluation *PEERS-ED* In this randomized controlled trial, the authors examined the role of congruent peer sleep educators and social support (PEERS-ED) in navigating Blacks seeking OSA care

Adults	8. Lack of racial/ethnic minorities in the field of sleep medicine	Implementation of training programs at the high school to faculty levels to increase minority representation in sleep medicine (eg, PRIDE, COMRADE & T32 programs Requirement for a specific quota of racial/ethnic minorities in the recruitment of future sleep specialists	Over the past decade, the authors' Behavioral Medicine & Sleep Disorders Research (PRIDE) program trained 62 under-represented minoritized (URM) scholars The Congruent Mentorship to Reach Academic Diversity (COMRADE) Summer Institute trained 22 URM scholars Through the T32 mentored-research training program, 12 URM postdoctoral fellows have been trained
Adults	9. Lack of research on epigenetic factors associated with sleep problems among children and adults	Implementation of multilevel research that explores links between individual and household/neighborhood factors with poor sleep Allocate funding to advance epigenetic studies on factors associated with poor sleep health.	In line with this specific policy, a genetic assessment component is included in the DORMIR study
	10. Lack of research on psychological resilience factors that are protective against factors that negatively affect sleep and CVD	Implementation of multilevel research that explores links among stress exposure and individual, social, cultural, and physical factors that affect sleep Allocate funding to advance research on sleep health resilience	Preliminary data from the authors' study on resilience factors, race/ethnicity, and sleep disturbance among diverse older women with hypertension suggest that resilience factors might be a more critical protective factor for sleep disturbance among diverse older women[20] Another study investigated the relationships among psychological resilience, peritraumatic distress, post-traumatic stress disorder (PTSD) and depression symptom severity, and sleep disturbances among survivors of the 2010 earthquake in Haiti 2 years later The findings support the importance of sleep in interventions aiming to improve the affected population's daily functioning[21]

IMPLEMENTING AND CONDUCTING COMMUNITY-BASED RESEARCH DURING CORONAVIRUS DISEASE 2019 THROUGH A DIGITAL HEALTH EQUITY FRAMEWORK

Overcoming sleep health disparities and inequities was already a challenge before the COVID pandemic, and became more challenging to address during the pandemic as sleep research laboratories, clinics, and practices had to adopt remote telehealth monitoring and treatment. Although telehealth monitoring and treatment proved to be initially successful in maintaining regular research and clinical operations in sleep medicine and research, it became apparent that minoritized communities did not benefit equally as white populations. The pandemic highlighted a digital divide between minoritized and nonminoritized communities and the need for a digital health equity model for sleep research and medicine.

Digital Divide

Novel approaches are needed to address the aforementioned barriers. Digital communication has become critical in remotely reaching participants and addressing key health care barriers. However, the demographic profile of Internet and social media users varies across platforms. Relying solely on digital communication may restrict the diversity of the participant pool. During the COVID-19 outbreak, 53% of Americans reported that the Internet was crucial. Nevertheless, lower-income Americans reported concerns about the digital divide and the digital homework gap. According to Pew Research Center, Black and Hispanic adults in the United States were less likely to have traditional computers and home broadband than non-Hispanic white populations. Americans with disabilities are less likely to own traditional computers and smartphones than those without them.[22] According to Pew Research Center, rural Americans have narrowed some digital gaps in the past decade by adopting digital technology. However, rural adults remain less likely than suburban adults to have home broadband and less likely than urban adults to own a smartphone, tablet computer, or traditional computer.[23]

This digital divide particularly affects older Black individuals. Less than half of Black adults over 65 year old use the Internet consistently. Instead, social network platforms like Facebook and Twitter may provide better opportunities to engage minoritized communities about sleep medicine and research as 61% of Black Internet users over 50 use these social network platforms.[24] However, the use of social network platforms is not consistent across all ages, and thus one cannot rely exclusively on social networks as the only method or media to engage individuals, especially among older minorities.[25] However, social network platform usage may be enhanced in this groups, and has proven particularly effective in conjunction with community-based efforts in the authors' work.[26]

Digital Health Equity and Inclusion in Sleep Medicine and Research

According to Healthy People 2020, health equity is achieved when everyone has the fair and just opportunity to attain their full health potential.[27,28] Digital health equity and inclusion, defined as the fair and just opportunity to engage with digital health tools to support good health outcomes, is equally crucial as health equity in sleep medicine and research.[29] To achieve comprehensive digital health equity and inclusion entails adequate digital health literacy, unrestricted access to digital resources, and the belief that digital solutions can be helpful for an individual's health.[30,31] Of the 3 factors, digital health literacy—the ability of an individual to obtain, process, and understand digital services and information–has proven to be one of the most important, as it can influence the other 2 factors, access of and belief in digital solutions.[30,31] To increase digital health literacy, technology solutions must be developed within a human-centric

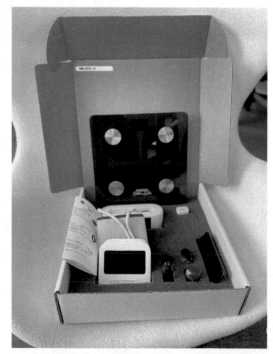

Fig. 2. The MILBox remote sleep and health monitoring solution.

Table 2
Implementing digital health equity framework in sleep research and medicine

Training	Training staff on processes and procedures for safely engaging, recruiting, and screening participants during the COVID-19 pandemic via various digital media such as video conference, phone, introductory e-mails, pamphlets, and word of mouth
Adaptation of study materials	Updated study manual, materials, and procedures manual (eg, data acquisition, processing, and storage using customized REDCap modules) to include staff and participant safety and preventive measures
Modification of study protocols	Profiles, PREDICT, ESSENTIAL, MOSAIC, and DORMIR performed entirely remotely, allowing the team to complete recruitment of participants even during the lockdown and work-from-home periods Profiles and PREDICT studies were conducted with participant sample sizes of 100 and 30, respectively, and recruitment targets were accomplished, even while enforcing social distancing and work-from-home periods in 2020, at the height of the COVID-19 response This remote methodology may be instrumental in reaching disadvantaged communities that would be otherwise unable or unwilling to participate in research in a clinical setting WIFI-enabled iPhones or iPads are provided to participants who do not have access to such devices or the Internet
Utilization of CSC	A CSC of health champions and/or community organizers from diverse backgrounds was created to act as an independent advisory group to the investigatory team The CSC provides guidance on community engagement, the use of technology, data sharing, and dissemination plans CSC key responsibilities are: 1. Provide feedback on modifying protocol procedures and feasibility and uptake of study procedures 2. Provide feedback on recruitment and retention procedures 3. Act as conduits and facilitators in onboarding and maintaining recruitment sites in the community 4. Assist with advertising and some public relations of the project 5. Provide concrete dissemination and implementation strategies to increase widespread community empowerment. The Community Steering Committee meets quarterly to discuss and provide guidance on all study related processes that impact participants and the community. The governance structure of the CSC consists of a chair, an Executive Secretary, and at least two other members. *Eligibility and selection of CSC.* To serve on the CSC, the member cannot have any conflict of interest with any of the collaborating or competing products or entities (devices, labs, firms, or other organizations) involved in the studies that constitute a potential conflict of interest. All CSC members are provided a nominal stipend for their efforts.

design focus, emphasizing better usability of digital devices and services and communicating tangible benefits of using these technology solutions to users. Using a human-centric design approach, the authors' team underwent a process of developing a remote health and sleep monitoring solution, The MIL BOX (see **Fig. 1**) to support 3 National Institutes of Health (NIH)-funded community-based projects (ESSENTIAL [R01HL142066], MOSAIC [NIH R01AG067523], and DORMIR [NIH R01HL152453], see **Table 1**) all aimed at investigating multilevel determinants of insufficient sleep

and its related heart and brain health consequences among Black and Latino populations **Fig. 2**.

In addition to creating The MIL Box, the authors also revamped their entire recruitment and retention strategy for minoritized participants during the COVID-19 pandemic to accommodate the new federal and state guidelines of social distancing to keep participants and staff engaged and safe (**Table 2**). Table 2 describes the authors' implementation of a digital health equity and inclusion framework across the research process and

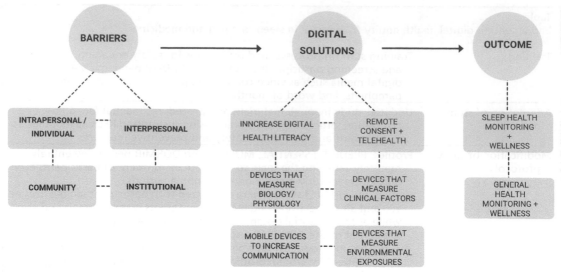

Fig. 3. Digital health equity and inclusion model.

Table 3
Digital health equity and inclusion model addresses research barriers

Phase of Research Process	Traditional Approaches	Barriers	Digital Health Equity and Inclusion Model
Engagement	Phone calls Field visits	Intrapersonal and psychosocial Time-consuming Low literacy Attitude Beliefs	Establishes stronger relationships Improves comprehension Reduces time
Recruitment	Community recruiters Field visits Community events	Interpersonal Mistrust Language Cultural	CSC Robust community engagement and recruitment program
Screening/consent	In-person contact	Institutional and systemic mistrust	Informed consent form cocreated alongside CSC for ultimate transparency Screening and consent process conducted over the phone for flexibility
Surveys	Filled out in person	Interpersonal Language Cultural differences Low literacy	All materials are translated Culturally trained and competent staff Raises cultural intelligence
Study execution and dissemination	In-person laboratory visits	Intrapersonal and psychosocial barriers Time-consuming Inconvenient Burdensome	Inclusive eligibility criteria focusing on minoritized groups Flexible operational hours 7-day home recording

journey, including training of staff, adaptation of study materials, modification of study protocols, and utilization of the CSC.

Revamping a Culturally Tailored Community Outreach Program to Meet the Challenges of the Coronavirus Disease 2019 Pandemic

In addition to implementing a digital health equity and inclusion model for sleep medicine and research, the authors revamped their culturally tailored community outreach program to meet the challenges of the COVID-19 pandemic. Guided by their mission to achieve sleep health equity and digital health equity and inclusion, throughout the COVID-19 pandemic the authors developed a culturally tailored community outreach program (COP) with several components to support the aforementioned NIH research projects: ESSENTIAL, MOSAIC and DORMIR. The focus of these studies is to investigate multilevel determinants of poor sleep among marginalized communities in the New York tristate and Florida. Outside of successfully executing the deliverables of the 3 projects, the authors' ultimate goal is to create a robust research and clinical infrastructure to enable and increase the inclusion of minoritized communities in research and clinical care. Increasing access to cost-effective digital health solutions is a critical mission of the authors' community-based research program (**Fig. 3**). Accordingly, the main objective of the authors' digital health equity and inclusion model is to leverage the latest digital technologies devices and innovations to measure multilevel factors that affect sleep and health among minoritized communities:

- Biological/physiological (eg, blood pressure, apnea hypopnea index, oxygen saturation, weight, and body composition)
- Behavioral (eg, sleep-wake patterns and physical activity)
- Clinical (eg, cognitive functioning, hemoglobin A1c [HbA1c], lipid profile, and inflammatory markers)
- Environmental (eg, temperature, humidity, carbon levels, and particulate matter)

Table 3 describes how together the authors' culturally tailored COP and digital health equity and inclusion model addressed intrapersonal, interpersonal, community, and institutional barriers to participating in sleep medicine and research. Specifically, the table describes significant barriers along 5 key processes in the research journey (engagement, recruitment, screening/consent, survey administration, and study execution and

dissemination) and highlights how key strategies in the culturally tailored COP and digital health equity and inclusion models addressed these barriers.

SUMMARY

The COVID-19 pandemic spotlighted and magnified long-standing sleep health disparities among minoritized communities in the United States, with worsening sleep health during the pandemic and restricted access to sleep medicine.[2] Increasing the participation of individuals from minoritized communities in sleep medicine and research is essential to reduce sleep health disparities. However, the current sleep medicine and research models are replete with intrapersonal/psychosocial, interpersonal, community and institutional/systemic barriers making participation difficult for minorities communities. The COVID-19 pandemic provided an opportunity to address these barriers through digital technology. Despite the promise of digital technologies to improve sleep medicine and research in minoritized communities, issues around lack of access to devices, low digital health literacy, and high cost of digital technologies may thwart plans to achieve equity in sleep medicine and research. Steeped in a community-based participatory research framework, the authors created a digital health equity model and remote health monitoring solution to address the aforementioned barriers. The authors have successfully incorporated this digital health equity model in all of their biomedical research projects, which helped them to overcome acute barriers to participation in sleep medicine and research caused by the pandemic, as well as long-term barriers around access. Utilizing a digital health equity model and strategy enabled the authors to overcome obstacles in recruitment while ensuring equal access to individuals from minoritized groups.

CLINICS CARE POINTS

- Utilize telemedicine and other technology tools to improve access to care for underrepresented groups facing transportation or other barriers to care. Remote patient monitoring can be an effective way to achieve this.
- Provide education materials in the patients' preferred language and format to ensure they understand the purpose and use of technology tools like sleep tracking applications, wearable devices, and Internet of things

(IoT) devices that capture bed environment data.

- Address cost and accessibility concerns related to technology tools and help patients identify resources and support to overcome these barriers.
- Respect cultural norms related to privacy and confidentiality when using technology tools like video conferencing, electronic health records, and IoT devices.
- Take into account the patient's technological literacy and comfort level when selecting and recommending technology tools.
- Provide clear instructions and support to help patients use technology tools effectively and troubleshoot any issues that arise, including IoT devices that capture bed environment data.
- Address any potential cultural barriers to using technology, such as concerns about the accuracy of technology tools, preference for in-person care, or discomfort with IoT devices that capture bed environment data.
- Utilize IoT devices that capture bed environment data to gather more accurate and detailed information about a patient's sleep environment and how it may impact his or her sleep health. This information can be particularly valuable for under-represented groups experiencing disparities in their sleep environment.
- Use these data to develop personalized sleep plans that address any issues related to a patient's sleep environment and to track the effectiveness of interventions over time.
- Use evidence-based guidelines and best practices to inform the selection and use of technology tools in sleep medicine, including IoT devices that capture bed environment data, while also being responsive to the patient's cultural needs and preferences.

POTENTIAL CONFLICTS OF INTEREST

The authors have no conflicts of interest to declare. This research was supported by funding from the NIH: K01HL135452, K07AG052685, R01AG072644, R01HL152453, R01MD007716, R01HL142066, R01AG067523, R01AG056031, and R01AG075007. The funding sources had no role in the study's design, conduct, analysis, or decision to submit the article for publication.

ACKNOWLEDGMENTS

The authors acknowledge the support of several funding agencies and the efforts of study staff, namely Kayla Taylor, Malik Ellington, Leo Landron, Clarence Locklear, Arlener Turner, PhD, and other interns and staff of the Center for Translational Sleep and Circadian Sciences (TSCS) and The Media and Innovation Lab at the University of Miami Miller School of Medicine, key and participants who all contributed to making the study successful. The authors are particularly grateful to the cochairs of TSCS's Community Steering Committee, Yolette Williams and Guithele Ruiz Nicolas, for connecting them with New York and South Florida communities and brokering these community relationships. All coauthors meet the criteria for authorship, including acceptance of responsibility for the scientific content of the paper. They have seen and agreed on the article's contents, and there is no financial conflict or conflicts of interest to report. They certify that the submission is the original work and is not under review at any other publication. J. Blanc and A.A. Seixas (corresponding authors) conceptualized the study and oversaw all aspects of the article. All other authors prepared tables and figures, helped to develop the scientific arguments, contributed to developing the scientific ideas and the discussion, and reviewed/edited the article.

REFERENCES

1. Cucinotta D, Vanelli M. WHO declares COVID-19 a pandemic. Acta Biomed 2020;91(1):157–60.
2. Lackland DT, Sims-Robinson C, Jones Buie JN, et al. Impact of COVID-19 on clinical research and inclusion of diverse populations. Ethn Dis 2020;30(3): 429–32.
3. Strully KW, Harrison TM, Pardo TA, et al. Strategies to address COVID-19 vaccine hesitancy and mitigate health disparities in minority populations. Front Public Health 2021;(9):645268.
4. Ballard EL, Gwyther LP, Edmonds HL. Challenges and opportunities: recruitment and retention of African Americans for Alzheimer disease research: lessons learned. Alzheimer Dis Assoc Disord 2010; 24(Suppl):S19–23.
5. Thakur N, Lovinsky-Desir S, Appell D, et al. Enhancing recruitment and retention of minority populations for clinical research in pulmonary, critical care, and sleep medicine: an official american thoracic society research statement. Am J Respir Crit Care Med 2021;204(3):e26–50.
6. Review of the literature: primary barriers and facilitators to participation in clinical research. National Institutes of Health. Available at: https://orwh.od.nih. gov/sites/orwh/files/docs/orwh_outreach_toolkit_ litreview.pdf. Accessed November 11-14, 2022.
7. Seixas AA, Trinh-Shevrin C, Ravenell J, et al. Culturally tailored, peer-based sleep health education and

social support to increase obstructive sleep apnea assessment and treatment adherence among a community sample of blacks: study protocol for a randomized controlled trial. Trials 2018;19(1):519.

8. Evans KR, Lewis MJ, Hudson SV. The role of health literacy on African American and Hispanic/Latino perspectives on cancer clinical trials. J Cancer Educ 2012;27(2):299–305.

9. Shah A, Macauley C, Ni L, et al. The relationship between attitudes about research and health literacy among African American and white (non-Hispanic) community dwelling older adults. J Racial Ethn Health Disparities 2022;9(1):93–102.

10. Lubetkin EI, Zabor EC, Isaac K, et al. Health literacy, information seeking, and trust in information in Haitians. Am J Health Behav 2015;39(3):441–50.

11. Richardson S, Lawrence K, Schoenthaler AM, et al. A framework for digital health equity. NPJ Digit Med 2022;5:119. https://doi.org/10.1038/s41746-022-00663-0.

12. Renzaho AM, Romios P, Crock C, et al. The effectiveness of cultural competence programs in ethnic minority patient-centered health care–a systematic review of the literature. Int J Qual Health Care 2013;25(3):261–9.

13. Al Shamsi H, Almutairi AG, Al Mashrafi S, et al. Implications of language barriers for healthcare: a systematic review. Oman Med J 2020;35(2):e122.

14. George S, Duran N, Norris K. A systematic review of barriers and facilitators to minority research participation among African Americans, Latinos, Asian Americans, and Pacific Islanders. Am J Public Health 2014;104(2):e16–31.

15. Ighodaro ET, Nelson PT, Kukull WA, et al. Challenges and considerations related to studying dementia in blacks/African Americans. J Alzheimers Dis 2017;60(1):1–10.

16. Seixas AA, Moore J, Chung A, et al. Benefits of community-based approaches in assessing and addressing sleep health and sleep-related cardiovascular disease risk: a precision and personalized population health approach. Curr Hypertens Rep 2020;22(8):52.

17. Blanc J, Nunes J, Williams N, et al. Sleep and health equity. Google Books.

18. Chung A, Jin P, Kamboukos D, et al. Out like a light: feasibility and acceptability study of an audio-based sleep aide for improving parent–child sleep health. Int J Environ Res Publ Health 2022;19(15):9416.

19. Oliveira BC, Vidal C, Pichardo Y, et al. 0621 Overcoming obstacles to recruitment and community engagement during COVID-19 and development of a digital community outreach program. Sleep 2022;45(Suppl 1):A272.

20. Blanc J, Seixas A, Donley T, et al. Resilience factors, race/ethnicity and sleep disturbance among diverse older females with hypertension. J Affect Disord 2020;271:255–61.

21. Blanc J, Spruill T, Butler M, et al. Is resilience a protective factor for sleep disturbances among earthquake survivors? Sleep 2019;42.

22. Atske S, Perrin A. Home broadband adoption, computer ownership vary by race, ethnicity in the U.S. Pew Research Center. Available at: https://www.pewresearch.org/fact-tank/2021/07/16/home-broadband-adoption-computer-ownersh ip-vary-by-race-ethnicity-in-the-u-s/. Accessed November 11-14, 2022.

23. Vogels EA. Some digital divides persist between rural, urban and Suburban America. Pew Research Center. Available at: https://www.pewresearch.org/fact-tank/2021/08/19/some-digital- divides-persist-between-rural-urban-and-suburban-america/. Accessed November 11-14, 2022.

24. Shearer E, Mitchell A. News use across social media platforms in 2020. Pew Research Center's Journalism Project. Available at: https://www.pewresearch.org/journalism/2021/01/12/news-use-across -social-media-platforms-in-2020/. Accessed November 11-14, 2022.

25. Smith A. Detailed demographic tables. Pew Research Center: Internet, science & tech. Available at: https://www.pewresearch.org/internet/2014/01/06/detailed-demographic-tables/. Accessed November 11-14, 2022.

26. Stout SH, Babulal GM, Johnson AM, et al. Recruitment of African American and non-Hispanic white older adults for Alzheimer disease research via traditional and social media: a case study. J Cross Cult Gerontol 2020;35(3):329–39.

27. Disparities, Healthy People.gov. Available at: https://www.healthypeople.gov/2020/about/foundation-health-measures/Disparities. Accessed November 11-14, 2022.

28. What is health equity? RWJF. Available at: https://www.rwjf.org/en/library/research/2017/05/what-is-health-equity-.html. Accessed November 11-14, 2022.

29. Digital health equity and COVID-19: the innovation curve cannot reinforce the social gradient of health. Duke Mobile App Gateway. Available at: https://www.mag.mobile.duke.edu/blog/2020/9/11/digital-health-equity-and-health-care-transformed-amid-covid-19. Accessed November 11-14, 2022.

30. Rodriguez JA, Clark CR, Bates DW. Digital health equity as a necessity in the 21st Century Cures Act era. JAMA 2020;323(23):2381–2.

31. Kaihlanen AM, Virtanen L, Buchert U, et al. Towards digital health equity - a qualitative study of the challenges experienced by vulnerable groups in using digital health services in the COVID-19 era. BMC Health Serv Res 2022;22(1):188.

Integrative Approach to Managing Obstructive Sleep Apnea

Kathleen R. Billings, MD[a,b,*], John Maddalozzo, MD[a,b]

KEYWORDS

- Obstructive sleep apnea • Integrative medicine • Complementary and integrative medicine
- Continuous positive airway pressure

KEY POINTS

- Conventional therapies for obstructive sleep apnea (OSA), including continuous positive airway pressure and oral appliances, offer the best opportunity for symptomatic improvement and reduction in OSA overall health impact.
- Integrative medicine brings conventional and complementary approaches together in a coordinated way.
- With rising obesity rates, weight loss and lifestyle programs seem to be the most favorable integrative methods to combine with conventional OSA therapies.
- Complementary and alternative approaches to OSA management are varied and, in conjunction with conventional methods, may offer some reduction in the apnea-hypopnea index (AHI).
- Studies of complementary and integrative management options alone have not demonstrated sustainable reductions in the AHI.

OVERVIEW

Obstructive sleep apnea (OSA) is a common disorder affecting 14% of men and 5% of women when defined by the apnea-hypopnea index (AHI) greater than 5 events/h and symptoms of daytime sleepiness.[1–3] Adult OSA is associated with several adverse effects if left untreated, including daytime sleepiness, reduced quality of life (QoL), increased cardiovascular morbidity and mortality, and increased risk of motor vehicle accidents.[4–7] The conventional treatment of OSA includes noninvasive options, that is, continuous positive airway pressure (CPAP) and dental appliances and invasive options, including a variety of surgical procedures aimed at addressing site-specific areas of upper airway obstruction. The goal of any treatment is reduction in sleep disruption and the AHI, with resultant improved overall health and QoL.

CONVENTIONAL TREATMENT APPROACHES AND OUTCOMES FOR OBSTRUCTIVE SLEEP APNEA

The gold standard treatment of OSA is CPAP.[1,8] CPAP is effective in preventing upper airway collapse, correcting oxyhemoglobin saturation, and reducing cortical arousals associated with apnea/hypopnea events. Despite improvements in mask design and flow technology to address issues with PAP mask tolerance, a large number of patients struggle to adhere to long-term PAP therapy.[9–11] Nonadherence rates with PAP therapy are

This article originally appeared in *Otolaryngologic Clinics of North America*, Volume 55 Issue 5, October 2022.
^a Division of Pediatric Otolaryngology-Head and Neck Surgery, Ann & Robert H. Lurie Children's Hospital of Chicago, 225 E Chciago Ave, Box #25, Chicago, IL, 60611, USA; ^b Department of Otolaryngology-Head and Neck Surgery, Northwestern University Feinberg School of Medicine, 675 N St Clair St, Chicago, IL, 60611, USA
* Corresponding author. Division of Otolaryngology-Head and Neck Surgery, Ann & Robert H. Lurie Children's Hospital of Chicago, 225 East Chicago Ave, Box #25, Chicago, IL 60611.
E-mail address: kbillings@luriechildrens.org

Sleep Med Clin 18 (2023) 269–275
https://doi.org/10.1016/j.jsmc.2023.05.011

reported to range from 20% to 40%, and patients with moderate to severe sleep apnea with poor compliance may continue to experience significant sequelae secondary to OSA.[12] With rising rates of OSA in adults related to increased rates of obesity and an aging population, both risk factors for OSA,[13] poor adherence to PAP therapy highlights the importance of a multifaceted approach in the care of patients with OSA.

Mandibular advancement devices (MADs), and other oral appliances, offer an alternative, noninvasive option for OSA management.[9] MADs consist of superior and inferior plates that are interconnected and work by displacing the mandible forward during sleep, thereby opening the posterior pharyngeal space. Kashida *and colleagues*[14] described MADs as a first-line therapy or alternative to PAP therapy in patients with mild to moderate OSA, and a second-line therapy for those with severe OSA who have failed PAP therapy. Reduction in the AHI and Epworth Sleepiness Scale (ESS) has been demonstrated with MADs, when compared with no interventions.[9,15,16] There are several side effects associated with MADs and close monitoring with a dentist specializing in sleep medicine is recommended, as the appliance may need to be replaced or adjusted over time with extended use.[9] Patients fitted with an oral appliance should undergo a polysomnogram (PSG) with the appliance in place after final adjustments to the fit have been performed. In addition, some patients may benefit from MAD use in conjunction with PAP treatment. Noninvasive options for OSA management are shown in **Box 1**.

A variety of surgical options to open the airway are available for the management of OSA. Carberry and colleagues[13] suggested that surgeries that target the anatomy of the upper airway could be a useful adjunct to improve the efficacy of other treatments such as CPAP and MADs. Clinical success for upper airway surgery is typically defined as a greater than 50% reduction in the AHI to less than 20 events/h, but the success rates of

surgery range from 5% to 78%.[17] Surgical options (**Box 2**) are varied and target patient-specific areas of upper airway obstruction, either alone or in combination with other procedures. The disadvantages of surgical procedures include their cost, varied and unpredictable efficacy, pain, infections, and anesthetic complications.[13] Surgical procedures may facilitate comfort with adjunctive CPAP use in some patients.

INTEGRATIVE TREATMENT APPROACHES AND OUTCOMES FOR OBSTRUCTIVE SLEEP APNEA

Complementary and integrative medicine (CIM) approaches are defined as a group of diverse medical and health care systems, practices, and products that are not presently considered to be part of conventional medicine.[18] The five subgroups of CIM therapies are shown in **Box 3**. Complementary interventions are used along with conventional treatments, whereas alternative approaches are used instead of conventional medicine. The term integrative refers to practice that includes two or more disciplines or distinct approaches to care.[19] Integrative health brings conventional and complementary approaches together in a coordinated way. As per web-based content,[20] integrative health emphasizes multimodal interventions, including combinations of conventional medicine, lifestyle changes, physical rehabilitation, psychotherapy, and complementary health approaches. The emphasis is on treating the whole person rather than one organ system. People who choose CIM are potentially seeking ways to improve their health and well-

---

Box 1
Noninvasive Obstructive Sleep Apnea Options

Noninvasive Obstructive Sleep Apnea Management

Continuous positive airway pressure

Mandibular advancement devices

Weight loss (dietary and exercise regimens)

Positional devices for sleep

Adjuvant nasal therapies (eg, nasal steroids)

Box 2
Surgical Options for Obstructive Sleep Apnea*

Surgical Obstructive Sleep Apnea Management

Tonsillectomy

Adenoidectomy

Uvulopalatopharyngoplasty (UPPP); modified or variant UPPP

Maxillomandibular advancement

Expansion sphincteroplasty

Lingual tonsillar reduction

Midline glossectomy

Transoral robotic surgery of tongue base reduction procedures

Hypoglossal nerve stimulator

*not comprehensive, other options for surgery available at discretion of treating physician

> **Box 3**
> **Five Categories of Complementary and Integrative Medicine Approaches**
>
> Complementary and Integrative Medicine Approaches
>
> Alternative medical systems (eg, acupuncture, Ayurveda)
>
> Mind–body interventions (eg, meditation)
>
> Biologically based therapies (eg, herbal supplements)
>
> Manipulative and body-based methods (eg, chiropractic therapy, osteopathic medicine)
>
> Energy therapies (eg, magnetic therapy)

being or to relieve symptoms associated with chronic illnesses or the side effects of conventional treatments. In the United States, the increased use of acupuncture, deep breathing exercises, massage therapy, naturopathy, and yoga were seen in adults between the years 2002 and 2007.[18]

Integrative Therapies for Obstructive Sleep Apnea

Epidemiologic studies have shown a strong association between excess weight and OSA in that most individuals with moderate to severe OSA also have an elevated body mass index.[21,22] Integrative therapies aimed at lifestyle changes and weight loss should play a role in managing obese patients with OSA, regardless of the conventional treatment being used. The pathophysiology of OSA, as it relates to obesity, can involve excess pharyngeal adipose tissue, which leads to airway narrowing, and excess abdominal wall and chest wall fat, which reduces lung volumes[21,23] A longitudinal prospective cohort study, the Wisconsin Sleep Disorder Study, found that weight loss of about 10% predicted a 26% reduction in the AHI.[21,24] Garvey and colleagues[25] suggested that for clinically significant and meaningful improvement in OSA, the weight loss goal should be at least 7% to 10%. Lifestyle modifications with reduced calorie intake and increased physical activity form the foundation of all weight loss interventions and have been demonstrated to result in weight-independent benefits in OSA.[26]

A randomized control trial (RCT) comparing the effectiveness of an intensive weight loss program for severe OSA in patients on CPAP showed a significant reduction in weight loss in the intervention group, when compared with the control group (received standard lifestyle recommendations).[1]

The AHI decreased more in the intervention group (−23.72 vs −9 events/h) at 3 months, but there was no difference between the groups at 12 months. There were improvements in the lipid profiles, glycemic control, and inflammatory markers in the intervention group, and the authors highlighted the importance of incorporating weight loss programs in the treatment of those with severe OSA on CPAP with the aim of improving their general health status.

Another study demonstrated the clinical importance of lifestyle modifications in addition to CPAP treatment in patients with OSA. Igelstrom and colleagues[27] performed an RCT comparing overweight patients with moderate–severe OSA who were assigned to a CPAP and behavioral sleep medicine (BSM) interventions targeting physical activity and eating behavior experimental group or a CPAP and advice about weight loss control group. There was a mean improvement in the AHI by 9.7 events/h in the experimental group, and 40% ($n = 14$) of patients in the experimental group had reduced severity of their OSA compared with 16.7% ($n = 6$, $P = .02$) in the control group. Despite improvements with BSM, the number of patients studied was small, and the sustainability of the impact of BSM on weight loss and AHI was not demonstrated in this 6-month trial. The authors commented that behavioral changes may not cure OSA but may be clinically relevant to the individual by reducing the disease severity and thereby the risk of comorbidities.

In Saunder and colleagues[21] review of surgical and nonsurgical weight loss for those with OSA, diet, physical activity, and behavioral modifications were described as the cornerstone of weight management. The authors cite a previous meta-analysis[28] suggesting that significant weight loss was observed with any low-carbohydrate or low-fat diet and that the best diet for any given patient was the one they could adhere to. Despite diet and weight loss interventions, many patients require additional interventions, such as anti-obesity medications and weight loss (bariatric) surgery.[21] Pharmaceuticals used for weight loss, and the range of bariatric surgery options and outcomes are well reviewed by the authors, although these additional options fall into conventional medicine approaches.

Integrative Medical Systems

Nonconventional CIM approaches, which can be used in the management of patients with OSA, include alternative medical systems, such as acupuncture and Ayurveda. Acupuncture originated in China thousands of years ago and has been used to treat a variety of maladies. Even today, it is one of the potential treatment options for those with chronic pain who are seen by the pain management services at many institutions. Evidence has shown that the effects of acupuncture include the release of serotonin from the caudal raphe nucleus and endogenous opioid systems[29,30] For those with OSA, the activation of these pathways stimulates upper airway motor neurons allowing for increased muscle tone in the area, thereby preventing pharyngeal collapse. Several studies have analyzed the utility of acupuncture in treating OSA.[29–31]

A meta-analysis evaluating the efficacy of acupuncture for OSA management included nine RCTs.[29] The cumulative analysis showed acupuncture significantly reduced the AHI in those with OSA, especially in moderate to severe cases. Results of the studies were not able to demonstrate a clinically significant threshold of AHI improvement and could not determine the curative effect of acupuncture for OSA treatment. The quality of evidence of included studies was mainly low to very low. One of the RCTs included in the meta-analysis was a study by Freire and colleagues.[30] The authors designed a randomized, placebo-controlled trial looking at the efficacy of treating moderate OSA with acupuncture. Patients enrolled in the study received acupuncture or sham acupuncture once a week for 10 weeks. A control group received no acupuncture. The sham group was stimulated with the same number of needles, but not in regions related to any acupoints, and the needles were not manipulated. The AHI and the number of respiratory events decreased significantly in the acupuncture group but not in the sham group. The sham group did not differ from the control group in any of the post-treatment PSG measurements. All the acupuncture patients had improved mental health scores on the posttreatment ESS and short form 36 (SF-36) questionnaires, and the authors noted the potential of acupuncture for a profound placebo effect.

Another RCT[31] studied the impact of acupuncture on OSA severity and blood pressure control in patients with hypertension ($n = 26$). The control group received sham acupuncture. The study did not demonstrate a reduction in OSA severity, daytime or nocturnal blood pressure, or QoL. The authors suggested that the number of treatment sessions were limited and may have impacted their results when compared with previous studies.

The utility of Chinese therapeutic massage (Tui Na) was investigated in a 1-year, single-blinded, randomized trial in 20 patients.[32] The treatment was given at multiple acupoints twice weekly for 10 weeks. The authors suggested that Tui Na of the neck and pharynx could affect muscles of the throat beneficially, thereby improving the stability of the upper airway. Some improvement in the AHI, QoL, sleep architecture, snoring intensity, and excessive daytime sleepiness was noted in their analysis.

Ayurveda is an ancient, holistic healing system developed over 1000 years ago in India. As per online content,[33,34] it is based on the concept of wellness and health being dependent on a manageable delicate balance between the spirit, mind, and body, with the goal to promote health and fight disease. These therapies seem to be targeted at some of the symptoms of sleep disturbances/OSA, such as cardiovascular issues, fatigue, headaches, and low productivity. The impact of Ayurveda on lowering the AHI in patients with OSA has not been specifically investigated.

Given the lack of existing evidence showing a long-term benefit to these therapies, they cannot be recommended as a primary treatment of OSA. As an adjunct to improving the comfort and QoL of patients, acupuncture and other complementary therapies are intriguing options, although the widespread availability of this resource in the United States is unclear and possibly limited in some regions.

Mind–Body Interventions

Mind–body interventions are the most common CIM therapies used in the United States and include meditation, relaxation, breathing techniques, T'ai chi and qigong (TCQ), hypnosis, and biofeedback.[35] T'ai Chi is a traditional Chinese martial art commonly used for health benefits. Qigong exercises form a basis for T'ai Chi and regulate mind, body, and breathing, and these exercises have been shown to improve fatigue, anxiety, depressive symptoms, and sleep disorders.[36] In an RCT performed in patients with mild to moderate OSA by Gokmen and colleagues,[36] an intervention group ($n = 25$) received TCQ training under a physiotherapist supervision along with a home exercise program, and the control group ($n = 25$) received a home exercise program. The intervention group was noted to have reduced AHI and daytime sleepiness, and improved subjective sleep quality when compared with the control group. Long-term outcomes were not analyzed.

Another study investigated the efficacy of mind–body (Baduanjin) exercise on self-reported sleep quality and QoL in elderly subjects with sleep disturbances.[37] These exercises involve coordinating one's breathing with physical movement slowly and gently, and the actions are less physically and cognitively demanding than other mind–body interventions. The authors noted an improved self-reported sleep quality in the intervention group, but no difference in QoL between the intervention and control groups. No AHI data were reported.

Biologically Based Therapies, Herbal and Dietary Supplements

As per Zhou and colleagues,[38] traditional Chinese medicine uses an overall therapeutic approach to treat and prevent inflammatory responses and oxidative stress with the aim of improving the patient's QoL. Traditional Chinese medicine offers a variety of active ingredients, which can act on targets simultaneously, rather than a single step Western medicine approach. The efficacy and safety of Chinese medicine for OSA was studied in a protocol for systematic review and meta-analysis by Bao and colleagues,[39] as a means of providing a reliable reference for the clinical application of Chinese medicine for OSA. The limitations of the analyses included differences in the doses of Chinese medicine used in the studies and the condition of the patient's disease.

The most common biologic products used to treat sleep disturbances, although not specifically OSA, include herbal tea, melatonin, chamomile, St. John's wort, lavender, and valerian.[40] Melatonin is a natural hormone produced and secreted by the pineal gland causing an increase in hypothalamus aminobutyric and serotonin. Increased secretion occurs during dark hours. Melatonin has been shown to help regulate the circadian rhythm and has been studied for treatment of delayed sleep phase syndrome and insomnia. Caution with use is recommended because of several drug interactions. Melatonin, chamomile, lavender, and valerian have a sedative effect and are not specifically recommended for the treatment of OSA.

The efficacy of oral dietary supplements has largely been based on subjective reports, and safety is assumed based on lack of reported adverse effects. Meoli and colleagues[41] discussed the efficacy of herbal lubricating nasal spray in their analysis. No significant objective difference in snoring intensity or frequency was seen, but bed partners reported a lessening in snoring intensity in 65% of patients. Physicians should question their patients about the use of these products, given the lack of published scientific evidence of objective benefits for these treatments in managing OSA. Patients should be counseled as to their potential risks and benefits, and the role of these remedies as a complement to conventional therapies not as an alternative should be reinforced.

Manipulative and Body-Based Methods

Manipulative and body-based practices focus primarily on the structures and systems of the body, including the bones and joints, the soft tissues, and the circulatory and lymphatic systems.[42,43] Practices include chiropractic and osteopathic manipulation, therapeutic massage, and yoga. Acupuncture and TCQ are also considered in this category. Intraoral myofascial therapy for the sphenopalatine ganglion (SPG) is widely used in osteopathic practice for the management of nasal obstruction, chronic rhinitis, and snoring. A proof-of-concept study to determine if manipulation of the SPG would improve pharyngeal stability in OSA was performed on nine subjects by Jacq and colleagues.[44] The findings of the study did not demonstrate efficacy of this treatment of OSA.

There is evidence that playing certain types of wind instruments was associated with improving the AHI and reducing the risk of developing OSA. In a systematic review by De Jong and colleagues,[45] the investigators suggested that by training and strengthening the muscles of the upper airway, patients could decrease airway collapsibility and effectively reduce progression and development of OSA. Instruments are accessible, inexpensive, and could be an adjunctive treatment of OSA, but the study suggested more validated studies were needed, as most of the existing literature did not report on the AHI of patients analyzed.

Energy Therapies

Energy treatments are aimed at healing imbalances in the energy fields purported to be in and around the human body. Examples of energy therapies include Reiki, a spiritual, vibrational healing practice, and healing touch, hands used to facilitate physical, emotional, mental, and spiritual health.[46] These therapies are used by some individuals for managing insomnia and fatigue. There specific use for OSA management has not been investigated.

SUMMARY

Conventional treatments of OSA, including CPAP, oral appliances, and various surgical interventions in appropriately selected patients, are the mainstay of OSA management. Particularly with the rising rates of obesity, integrative approaches to improve weight loss and lifestyle habits are essential to managing patients with OSA to aid in achieving longer term success. CIM therapies, as part of an integrative approach to treating OSA, may result in improving symptoms of sleep disturbances and QoL, but they may not be associated with sustainable reductions in the AHI when used alone. As more and more patients seek CIM treatments, physicians should be aware of their role and utility in treating patients with OSA.

DISCLOSURES/CONFLICTS

The authors have no disclosures or conflicts of interest.

REFERENCES

1. Lopez-Padros C, Salord N, Alves C, et al. Effectiveness of an intensive weight-loss program for severe OSA in patients undergoing CPAP treatment: randomized controlled trial. J Clin Sleep Med 2020; 16(4):503–14.
2. Peppard PE, Young T, Palta M, et al. Increased prevalence of sleep-disordered breathing in adults. Am J Epidemiol 2013;177(9):1006–14.
3. Gavrey JF, Pengo MF, Drakatos P, et al. Epidemiological aspects of obstructive sleep apnea. J Thorac Dis 2015;7(5):920–9.
4. MacKay S, As Carney, Catcheside PG, et al. Effect of multilevel upper airway surgery vs medical management on the apnea-hypopnea index and patient-reported daytime sleepiness among patients with moderate or severe obstructive sleep apnea: the SAMS randomized clinical trial. JAMA 2020; 324(12):1168–79.
5. Kie C, Zhu R, Tian Y, et al. Association of obstructive sleep apnoea with the risk of vascular outcomes and all-cause mortality: a meta-analysis. BMJ Open 2017;7(12):e013983.
6. Patil SP, Ayappe IA, Caples SM, et al. Treatment of adult obstructive sleep apnea with positive airway pressure: an American Academy of Sleep Medicine systematic review, meta-analysis, and GRADE assessment. J Clin Sleep Med 2019;15(2):301–34.
7. Tregear S, Reston J, Schoelles K, et al. Obstructive sleep apnea and risk of motor vehicle crash: a systematic review and meta-analysis. J Clin Sleep Med 2009;5(6):573–81.
8. McDaid C, Duree KH, Griffin SC, et al. A systematic review of continuous positive airway pressure for obstructive sleep apnea-hypopnoea syndrome. Sleep Med Rev 2009;13(6):427–36.
9. Suurna MV, Frieger AC. Obstructive sleep apnea: Non-positive airway pressure treatments. Clin Geriatr Med 2021;37:429–44.
10. Rotenberg BW, Marariu D, Pang KP. Trends in CPAP adherence over twenty years of data collection: a flattened curve. J Otolaryngol Head Neck Surg 2016;45:43.
11. Sawyer AM, Gooneratne NS, Marcus CL, et al. A systematic review of CPAP adherence across age groups: clinical and empiric insights for developing CPAP adherence interventions. Sleep Med Rev 2011;15(6):343–56.
12. Kent D, Stanley J, Aurora N, et al. Referral of adults with obstructive sleep apnea for surgical consultation: an American Academy of Sleep Medicine systematic review, meta-analysis, and GRADE assessment. J Clin Sleep Med 2021;17(12):2507–31.
13. Carberry JC, Amatoury J, Eckert DJ. Personalized management approach for OSA. Chest 2018; 153(3):744–55.
14. Kashida CA, Littner MR, Morgenthaler T, et al. Practice parameters for the indications for polysomnography and related procedures: an update for 2005. Sleep 2005;28(4):499–521.
15. Blanco J, Zamarron C, Abeleira Pazos MT, et al. Prospective evaluation of an oral appliance in the treatment of obstructive sleep apnea syndrome. Sleep Breath 2005;9:20–5.
16. Petri N, Svanholt P, Solow B, et al. Mandibular advancement appliance for obstructive sleep apnea: results of a randomized placebo-controlled trial using parallel group design. J Sleep Res 2008;17:221–9.
17. Dorrity J, Wirtz N, Frymovich O, et al. Genioglossal advancement, hyoid suspension, tongue base radiofrequency, and endoscopic, partial midline glossectomy for obstructive sleep apnea. Otolaryngol Clin North Am 2016;49(6):1399–414.
18. Sood A, Narayanan S, Wahner-Roedler DL, et al. Use of complementary and alternative medicine treatments by patients with obstructive sleep apnea hypopnea syndrome. J Clin Sleep Med 2007;3(6):575–9.
19. Frish NC, Rabinowitsch D. What's in a definition? Holistic nursing, integrative health care, and integrative nursing: report of an integrated literature review. J Holist Nurs 2019;37(3):260–72.
20. Complementary, alternative, or integrative health: what's in a name?. Available at: www.nccih.nih.gov. Accessed January 30 2022.
21. Saunders KH, Igel LI, Tchang BG. Surgical and nonsurgical weight loss for patients with obstructive sleep apnea. Otolaryngol Clin North Am 2020;53: 409–20.
22. Young T, Peppard PE, Taheri S. Excess weight and sleep-disordered breathing. J Appl Physiol 1985; 99(4):1592–9.
23. Joosten SA, Hamilton GS, Naughton MT. Impact of weight loss management in OSA. Chest 2017; 152(1):194–203.
24. Peppard PE, Young T, Palta M, et al. Longitudinal study of moderate weight change and sleep-disordered breathing. JAMA 2000;284(23):3015–21.

25. Garvey WT, Garber AJ, Mechanik JI, et al. American association of clinical endocrinologists and American College of Endocrinology position statement on the 2014 advanced framework for a new diagnosis of obesity as a chronic disease. Endocr Pract 2014;20(9):977–89.

26. Tham KW, Ching Lee P, Lim CH. Weight management in obstructive sleep apnea: medical and surgical options. Sleep Med Clin 2019;14:143–53.

27. Igelstrom H, Asenlof P, Emtner M, et al. Improvement in obstructive sleep apnea after a tailored behavioral sleep medicine intervention targeting healthy eating and physical activity: a randomized controlled trial. Sleep Breath 2018;22:653–61.

28. Johnston BC, Kanters S, Bandayrei K, et al. Comparison of weight loss among named diet programs in overweight and obese adults: a meta-analysis. JAMA 2014;312(9):923–33.

29. Wang L, Xu J, Zhan Y, et al. Acupuncture for obstructive sleep apnea (OSA) in adults: a systematic review and meta-analysis. Biomed Res Internat 2020;ID6972327:1–10.

30. Friere AO, Sugai GCM, Chrispin FS, et al. treatment of moderate obstructive sleep apnea syndrome with acupuncture: a randomized, placebo-controlled pilot trial. Sleep Med 2007;8:43–50.

31. Silva MV, Lustosa TC, Arai VJ, et al. Effects of acupuncture on obstructive sleep apnea severity, blood pressure control and quality of life in patients with hypertension: a randomized controlled trial. J Sleep Res 2020;29:e12954.

32. Lu CN, Friedman M, Lin HC, et al. Alternative therapy for patients with obstructive sleep apnea/hypopnea syndrome: a 1-year, single-blind, randomized trial of Tui Na. Altern Ther Health Med 2017;23(4): 16–24.

33. Ayurveda for sleep apnea: natural remedies to cease snoring and ensure a deep slumber. Available at: www.netmeds.com. Accessed February 19 2022.

34. 5 Ayurvedic remedies for sleep apnea. Available at: www.shankara.com. Accessed February 19 2022.

35. Wahbeh H, Elsas SM, Oken BS. Mind-body interventions: applications in neurology. Neurology 2008; 70(24):2321–8.

36. Gokman GY, Akkoyunlu ME, Kilic L, et al. The effect of T'ai Chi and Qigong training on patients with obstructive sleep apnea: a randomized controlled study. J Altern Complement Med 2019;25(3): 317–25.

37. Fan B, Song W, Zhang J, et al. The efficacy of mind-body (Baduanjin) exercise on self-reported sleep quality and quality of life in elderly subjects with sleep disturbances: a randomized controlled trial. Sleep Breath 2020;24:696–701.

38. Zhou M, Liang Q, Pei Q, et al. Chinese herbs medicine Huatan Huoxue prescription for obstructive sleep apnea hypopnea syndrome as complementary therapy: a protocol for a systematic review and meta-analysis. Medicine 2020;99:e21070.

39. Bao JL, Gao X, Han YB, et al. Efficacy and Safety of Chinese medicine for obstructive sleep apnea. Medicine 2021;100(3):1–4.

40. Gooneratne NS. Complementary and alternative medicine for sleep disturbances in older adults. Clin Geriatr Med 2008;24(1):121–viii.

41. Meoli AL, Rosen CL, Kristo D, et al. Nonprescription treatments of snoring or obstructive sleep apnea: an evaluation of products with limited scientific evidence. Sleep 2003;26(5):619–24.

42. Manipulative and body-based practice: an overview. Available at: www.healthyplace.com. Accessed February 6 2022.

43. Jacq O, Arnulf I, Similowski T, et al. Upper airway stabilization by osteopathic manipulation of the sphenoplatine ganglion versus sham manipulation in OSAS patients: a proof-of-concept, randomized, crossover double-blind, controlled study. Complement Altern Med 2017;17(546):1–10.

44. De Jong JC, Maroda AJ, Camacho M, et al. The impact of playing a musical instrument on obstructive sleep apnea: a systematic review. Ann Otol Rhinol Laryngol 2020;129(9):924–9.

45. What is energy medicine?. Available at: www.nm. org. Accessed February 6 2022.

Challenges of Applying Automated Polysomnography Scoring at Scale

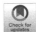

Diego Alvarez-Estevez, PhD

KEYWORDS

- Polysomnography • Automatic analysis • Performance assessment • Scalability challenges
- Artificial intelligence

KEY POINTS

- Automatic polysomnography analysis can greatly benefit diagnostic quality and efficiency of sleep disorders.
- Performance assessment of associated technology has multiple layers and is complicated to evaluate.
- Challenges remain in a number of areas, including assessment in varying populations, domain adaptation, inference interpretability, privacy and ethical safeguarding, or integration into existing clinical infrastructures.
- Recent developments in computer science and artificial intelligence are closing the gap for overcoming some of the challenges. They also have the potential to advance clinical knowledge in the field.
- The ultimate aim is to assist the clinical expert, who should retain control and be responsible for the final decision, to guarantee an optimal patient care.

INTRODUCTION

Polysomnography (PSG) is the standard diagnostic tool for a number of sleep disorders. It is a comprehensive test that records diverse neurophysiological data with a typical duration of more than 8 to 10 hours, if performed in a clinical setting, or longer, if performed in ambulatory conditions. The standard setup includes recording of several electroencephalographic (EEG), electrooculographic, electrocardiographic, electromyographic (EMG), or respiratory activity. Clinical guidelines are organized around specific sets of rules for the characterization of sleep and the scoring of related arousal, cardiac, movement, and respiratory events.[1]

PSG review is traditionally assessed visually by clinical experts but clinician time is both costly and scant. In addition, PSG generate vast amounts of complex data, making scoring difficult and increasing the likelihood of mistakes and interpretation variability.[2–4] Consequently, PSG scoring is one of the most time-consuming and expensive tasks in the day-to-day running of a sleep center. The situation is aggravated by the increasing demand for sleep studies, driven by last clinical findings and the general public awareness, which represents a challenge for the already congested sleep centers.

The development of automatic scoring algorithms should help reduce scoring times and enhance production rates. These systems also have the potential to improve the quality of diagnosis because computers produce deterministic, and hence repeatable, outputs. Literature, in fact,

Center for Information and Communications Technology Research (CITIC), Universidade da Coruña, 15071 A Coruña, Spain
E-mail address: diego.alvareze@udc.es

Sleep Med Clin 18 (2023) 277–292
https://doi.org/10.1016/j.jsmc.2023.05.002

is rich with examples of automated methods that focus on different areas related to PSG scoring. From first attempts back in the 1970s,[5,6] production began to flourish at the beginning of the twenty-first century,[7,8] peaking considerably in the last years in parallel with advances in artificial intelligence (AI) and the related subfield deep learning in particular.[9–11] **Fig. 1** shows the annual growth in publications on the subject of automatic PSG scoring based on a PubMed search using a combination of the terms *automatic, computer analysis, artificial intelligence, machine learning, deep learning, PSG,* and *sleep.* Today, new advances are being released on almost a daily basis, which makes it even difficult to keep track of the latest developments.

However, despite the recent scientific advances and promising man–machine validation results reported in some of the studies, uptake of automatic scoring systems in the clinical setting remains low.[9,12]

This article reviews current trends, challenges, and future directions related to the at-scale adoption of automatic PSG analysis. It should be noticed that the main focus thus concerns PSG scoring, whereas the role of computer analysis in sleep medicine can certainly be expanded to a number of additional subareas and diagnostic tools. Similarly, it is worth clarifying that the term *automatic analysis* is used throughout this text to refer to all computer-based scoring approaches, regardless of the technique used. Where appropriate, more precise terminology is used, particularly in relation to prominent techniques of AI and the subfields of machine learning (ML) and deep learning (DL). Regardless, it is beyond the scope of this text to enter the discussion of what makes a particular algorithm to fall into one or other of these categories. The

interested reader is referred to standard textbooks on the topic for further information.[13] Finally, in light of the rapid developments in the field, readers are also referred to several excellent reviews that have been recently published on more specific subtopics.[9,14,15]

CALIBRATING EXPECTATIONS: WHAT IS THE GOAL OF AUTOMATIC POLYSOMNOGRAPHY ANALYSIS?

Before addressing the challenges surrounding the application of automatic PSG analysis at scale, it is necessary to understand the main purpose of these systems and related expectations. Examining the question is closely linked to evaluation of the related performance. However, what does *performance* in the context of automatic PSG analysis actually mean? The specific qualification can take different forms depending on the context, which conditions the choice of appropriate metrics for objective quantification on each case. Thus, rather than with a single definition, performance assessment can be better approached as a multidimensional construct comprising numerous components (**Fig. 2**).

Some basic ideas have been pointed out during the introductory section, for example, in reference to the necessity of improving the scoring speed to lower down the associated reviewing costs. In this regard, a regular computer is today sufficiently powerful to complete a full PSG analysis in minutes. Repeatable outputs are also desirable, in contrast to outcome variability and scoring mistakes due to the human factor. Nonconventional approaches aside, such as quantum computing, it stands to reason that repeatability is also guaranteed by the deterministic nature of today's "classic" computers.

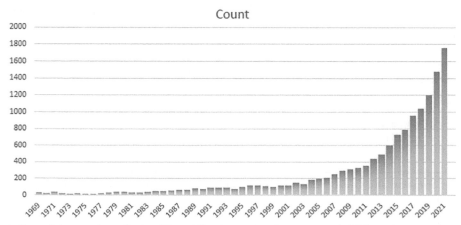

Fig. 1. Evolution of the number of scientific publications related to automatic PSG scoring per year.

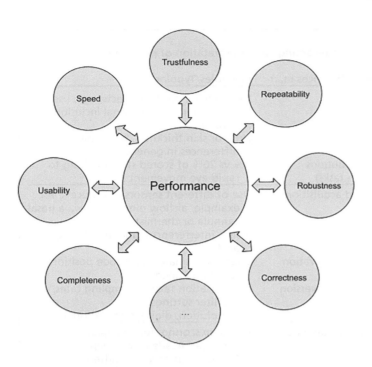

Fig. 2. Performance assessment of automatic PSG scoring as a multidimensional approach.

Other components of the performance ecosystem depicted in **Fig. 2** perhaps deserve more discussion. One potentially controversial issue regards dealing with the uncertainty inherent to the domain of PSG scoring, which arises questions on how to best evaluate the reliability or "correctness" of outputs in the absence of an objective, well-established, validation standard, or "ground truth."

THE PROBLEM OF RELIABILITY ASSESSMENT IN AUTOMATIC POLYSOMNOGRAPHY SCORING

One major challenge associated with automatic PSG scoring is the absence of an irrefutable standard reference against which to compare the output. That is, in contrast with other disciplines, there is no true gold standard, and traditionally the only available reference has been human scoring.[16] Even the most experienced scorers, however, are subject to commit mistakes and inconsistences, for example, by fatigue or mood swings. Subjective ratings are also affected by personal bias. As a result, rescoring by the same PSG expert will inevitably lead to slight variations (intraexpert variability). Variations will likely be greater when recordings are scored by different experts (interrater variability),[17] and even more, in general, among experts from different backgrounds or centers (intercenter variability).[18–24]

Intuitively, differences among subject demographics and associated monitoring conditions also modulate the effective intraexpert and interexpert variability levels (**Table 1**). The reference human agreement levels, therefore, depend to a certain extent on the characteristics of the local dataset used for evaluation. Hence, as each study uses its own data and analysis settings, rather than a single reference value, one can at best try to approximate plausible ranges by extrapolation from different works in the related literature. Notably, the reference human agreement levels also vary according to the specific PSG scoring task being evaluated.[17,21,25–27]

Although there is evidence that guidelines for the standardization of the scoring procedures[1,29] and periodic training[25,26,30–33] can limit the effects of variability, reliability assessment of automatic scoring is hindered by existence of various and unavoidable uncertainty sources.[22]

Validation of automatic scoring approaches has traditionally been problematic due to limitations of the available references and datasets. Data would be local and generally involve small, homogeneous, and/or underrepresented populations rated by single scorers.[7,8,11,34] Results are therefore not generalizable, and methods are often biased toward specific (and sometimes even optimistic) cases. The typical validation scenario would compare the output of a computer algorithm with manual scoring produced by a single human expert, claiming good performance by showing (almost) perfect agreement. This practice, however, introduces bias toward a given expert or reference dataset.

Comparing outputs against the scoring of multiple experts might be a preferable choice.[3,21,24,33,35,36]

Table 1
Different sources of variability affecting the recording and interpretation of polysomnography data

Category	Subcategory (differences in...)	Examples/Typologies
Source populations	Subject conditions	Diseased vs healthy subjects, age, use of medication, or additional inclusion criteria
	Physiology	Skull or skin thickness, anatomical differences in general
	Frequency distributions (classification tasks)	5% vs 20% of scored stages belong to rapid eye movement sleep
Recording and/or acquisition methods	Monitoring and acquisition conditions	Use of different sensors/transducers, for example, airflow monitoring via a nasal cannula or thermistor
		Noise, interferences, and monitoring artifacts
	Setup, montage, calibration	Channel mismatch, electrode positions, resulting impedances
	Analog to digital conversion	Amplification factors, sampling rates, prefilter settings
		Bit resolution, digital storage format
Data interpretation	Reference scoring standards	For sleep scoring, for example, American Academy of Sleep Medicine criteria (and different versions) vs Rechtschaffen and Kales criteria
		Use of different definitions of hypopnea, and so forth
	Intrascorer subjectivity	Tiredness, stress, general mood
	Interscorer subjectivity	Subjective interpretation of the same phenomena by 2 different persons, different training and/or experience, use of different ad hoc rules

Adapted from Alvarez-Estevez et al.[28]

This, in addition, makes it possible to obtain a database-specific baseline for the interexpert variability that can be used for human–machine evaluations. Unfortunately, the availability of multiscored validation benchmarks is very limited. The development of a sufficiently large and heterogeneous database, furthermore if scored by multiple experts, is a costly process subject to numerous technical and ethical issues.[3,37] Performing validation using multiple, heterogeneous databases is also important for testing the actual generalization capabilities of automatic scoring models. This topic will be discussed in detail in the next section.

An additional challenge is that in most validation studies, related methods and data, are privative, which prevents replication and objective comparison among different approaches. The absence of standardized validation procedures adds even more difficulty because each study uses its own metrics and methods for performance analysis.[22]

Living in the era of Big Data, the trend is progressively changing. Method source code sharing on publicly accessible repositories is increasingly becoming the norm. Data-generation capacity is growing exponentially, and challenges aside, an increasing number of benchmark databases are being made available online.[38,39] One such initiative involves the creation of a large gold standard dataset in which international expert scorers will identify relevant leg movement activity in EMG traces. Resulting data are expected not only to contribute to further understanding of related interrater reliability but also to inform future updates to little or ill-defined constructs, such as baseline EMG levels, and be useful for the development and validation of leg movement detection algorithms.[40]

Still, research and development efforts are required in light of the highlighted limitations. An important hypothesis behind the use of (semi-automatic) scoring is that it can help neutralize intraexpert and interexpert variability.[22] Addressing these effects and enhancing interdatabase generalization capabilities are active areas of research in the field.

INTERDATABASE GENERALIZATION AND DOMAIN ADAPTATION

The validation of automatic PSG scoring systems is hindered by numerous factors, including the multiple sources of variability summarized in **Table 1**.[28] One recent study discusses an alternative classification in terms of associated aleatoric and epistemic uncertainty.[33]

Although most of variability sources affect both, human-based and computer-based scoring, the latter is particularly influenced by technical challenges related to specifics of the recording hardware, the digitalization procedure, or the frequency distribution of the target domain classes in the training dataset. As a result, automatic algorithms tend to have difficulties sustaining their results beyond the original testing scenario (*source domain*) and experience a drop in performance when evaluated on unseen external data (*target domain*), even if concerning the same target task.[28] Effectively, data variability between different sleep datasets, each subject to specific conditions, leads to *domain shift*, making it easy for automatic scoring systems that were developed and/or tested on single-source data to over-fit to the particular source domain conditions. This is not particular to automatic PSG scoring but regards a known problem in ML referred to as the *domain adaptation*.

Driven by the growing data and benchmarking availability, one particularly active area of research in the recent years involves the problem of interdatabase generalization problem. A taxonomy-based classification of different approaches is provided in **Table 2**.

The generalization performance of algorithms (referred to as *learning models*, or simply *models* in the rest of this section as per standard ML terminology) has traditionally been estimated using single-source data, that is, data from a specific reference database. These data are typically split into separate training, validation, and testing subsets, with the first 2 used for model development and parameterization and the third set aside used to assess generalization. Alternatively, the source dataset can be partitioned using different variants of *k*-fold cross-validation, leading to *k* disjoint testing iterations of above-described train/validation/testing procedure.[41] Until recently, and still today, much of the related studies involving validation of PSG scoring algorithms used this approach.[8,15,42–51] Such process, however, does not involve *domain shift*, and hence does not constitute valid proof of interdatabase generalization. Several other approaches can be found in the literature that involve multiple independent datasets, however, in which the model is individually retrained or reparametrized *from scratch* on each of the datasets, or, alternatively, in which all datasets are split together using similar *local* or *in-domain* validation techniques.[14,52–56] Again, because the models are never tested on unseen external datasets, those procedures neither offer true proof of generalization.

Direct transfer is the scenario in which model performance is tested using fully external, unseen datasets. As mentioned, several studies have applied this setup showing that model development using single-source dataset usually experience a significant drop in performance.[28,34,57–64] The most straightforward way to overcome this problem is to increase the size and heterogeneity of training data by having the model learn from several datasets all at once.[65] This approach, however, has its own disadvantages,[28] for which alternative procedures have been proposed. For example, in past studies, we have proposed the use of an ensemble-based approach integrating local models.[23] One recent study showed that generalization capabilities can be enhanced by learning from the expert consensus, which is possible when multilabeled data are available (ie, recordings scored separately by multiple independent experts).[66] Another recent study suggested the use of alternative methods for inserting knowledge from multiple experts as a better approach.[67]

Under the common term of *transfer learning*, we can group a number of approaches that share the general idea of reusing knowledge or preparameterization acquired in the context of a source domain and transfer it to a different, yet related, context.[68] The idea of developing a preliminary model, using one or several datasets, and then *fine-tuning* certain parts, using data from another set of independent datasets, has been applied to automatic PSG scoring in recent studies.[61,66,69–79]

Most of the machine-learning approaches use labeled data from both source and target domain during the training process. However, as discussed in the previous section, because labeling has to be performed by human scorers, the procedure is expensive and scarcely scalable. *Semi-supervised domain adaptation* involves a limited set of labeled training data from external datasets, and examples can be found applied to automatic sleep staging.[71,72] One further step consists in using unlabeled data for model adaptation leading to *unsupervised domain adaptation*. Regardless, one common idea is the use of different levels of intermediate information to readjust the internal parameters of the model to increase robustness to

Table 2
Classification of automatic sleep scoring design and evaluation strategies in the context of interdatabase generalization and domain adaptation

Source dataset(s)	Intermediate independent dataset(s)	External target dataset(s)	Proof of interdatabase generalization	Nomenclature	Sub-variants
For model training or parametrization	–	No	No	Local or in-domain validation	• Train/validation/ test partitioning • K-fold validation
	Full model and/or data retraining	No	No	Learning from scratch	• Train/validation/ test partitioning • K-fold validation
	–	Only for testing	Yes	Direct transfer	–
	Part of the model or data	No	Limited	Transfer learning	• Model fine-tuning • Semisupervised domain adaptation • Unsupervised domain adaptation
	Part of the model or data	Only for testing	Yes		

domain shift variations. The literature describes several unsupervised domain adaptation approaches, again, applied to sleep stage classification. These can be further categorized as discrepancy-based or adversarial-based approaches. The first group attempts to minimize the distance between source and target domains by applying a learned transformation operation.[69,78] Adversarial learning uses competitive neural networks to promote the emergence of features that are both discriminative for the main learning task and indiscriminative with respect to the cross-domain shift.[75–77,79]

Importantly, all the above approaches use more or less information from intermediate datasets to transfer learning of some sort. Therefore, proof of actual generalization to totally unseen data remains uncertain. True interdatabase generalization setups work with completely independent datasets in a direct-transfer setting. The recent study of Abou-Jaude and colleagues is an example of transfer learning applied to automatic sleep staging that uses source and intermediate datasets for model development with additional testing on completely independent target scenario.[70]

DID AUTOMATIC SCORING ALREADY ACHIEVE (OR SURPASS) RELIABILITY OF HUMAN SCORING?

Sleep staging is by far the most-studied feature of automatic PSG analysis, and there is a growing wave of opinion that sufficient evidence now exists to show that reliability of machine-based scoring is on par,[16,24] or nearly performs as well as human experts[9,80] in this task. Other PSG analysis subdomains have also been studied; however, the accumulation of more evidence is probably needed in these cases for similar debates to be sustained. Full PSG analysis systems including arousals, respiratory events, and periodic leg movements have also been proposed in the past.[21,35,59,81,82] Comprehensive evaluation of their scoring reliability, however, remains limited.[24] Much remains thus to be done before "completeness" can be ticked off the list of pending items for achievement of full automatic PSG analysis at scale (see **Fig. 2**).

Regardless, several recent studies have suggested that automatic PSG scoring may already outperform expert humans in certain tasks.[24,36,54,66,83,84] The statement perhaps deserves a more detailed discussion.

The common experimental basis for the previous claim relies in the use of a pool of different experts, observing that the evaluated automatic algorithm can obtain slightly better agreement when compared one-to-one with each of the involved human experts. The reference model for that purpose is the expert consensus (usually based on a majority-voting approach) applied to all experts but one (leaving-one-out expert consensus). In other words, the output of the automatic algorithm is able to resemble the unbiased consensus more closely in comparison to the individual human expert. Although this result provides unequivocal proof of good (possibly good enough) automatic scoring reliability, it may not necessarily mean that the model has outperformed humans. Factoring that human scoring is the only available reference, it is difficult to envision performance beyond the limits set by the reference itself.

It is important to note that all the scoring algorithms analyzed in the above studies were developed using supervised ML.[41] In other words, the internal parameters or "weights" of the model were optimized to minimize output error with respect to the set of learning examples annotated, precisely, by human experts. As discussed in "The problem of reliability assessment in automatic polysomnography scoring" section, human scoring is nevertheless affected by imprecision due to different sources of variability. Hence, when provided with sufficient quantities of heterogeneous learning data, an algorithm trained in this manner would logically face variability by converging to average decisions.

The use of consensus as reference, however, is nothing but an ad hoc construct based on the idea that a consistent majority of agreeing experts exists. Remarkably, different studies in the context of sleep staging have shown that ambiguity seems to be the rule rather than the exception. Furthermore, overall agreement seems to be inversely proportional to the number of experts involved.[22,24] Intrinsic to the idea of consensus (or majority voting) is also that the opinion of all human scorers is equally valid. Individual deviations, thus, whether they represent the majority or not, do not necessarily correlate with the quality of the associated scoring. There are, however, no clear formulas to discern whose opinion represent the best reference in a group of human experts.

In absence of a better reference, it seems that there is no choice but to accept the limitations. The maximum aspiration for any automatic analysis software should thus to behave "as one expert more." Regardless, computer analysis can prove useful tools for characterization of the underlying uncertainty and the improvement of the diagnostic process.[16,24,33] One additional interesting possibility in this regard is the use of human–machine collaboration resulting in different forms of semiautomatic scoring. Several studies in the context of sleep staging have shown that baseline inter-rater agreement can be improved by applying different levels of expert supervision to an initial round of automatic scoring.[2,27,35,85–88] Similar results have been observed for other PSG scoring subtasks,[27,35] and some studies have even reported considerable time gains compared with manual analysis.[2,27,85,86] Full supervision, however, is probably unnecessary, and focus should rather be limited to examination of the most ambiguous recording periods.[24,85,89] For this purpose, the use of computer-assisted recording quality screening mechanisms have been found to significantly reduce the number of epochs that require human inspection.[90] Semiautomatic scoring could also be seen as an interesting intermediate step toward widespread adoption of full automatic systems. It can be useful for building confidence and trust among human experts and increase uptake in clinical practice.

TRUSTFULNESS, ACCOUNTABILITY, INTERPRETABILITY, AND TRANSPARENCY

One key aspect for the general acceptance and successful large-scale integration of automatic analysis in the clinical setting (which is extensible to many other critical domains) is the ability to build trust among end users. No matter how many metrics or validation studies may support its "general good operability," the presence of variability and uncertainty will inevitably trigger the necessity of further in-depth inspection in ambiguous cases. The intrinsically skeptic human will always demand traceability and justification of the generated system outputs. Automatic scoring algorithms must therefore offer accountability and interpretability.

One challenge related to interpretability is that it usually comes along with a certain toll on the associated accuracy. In the machine-learning literature this is known as "the accuracy-interpretability trade-off."[91] Some early approaches to interpretability in automatic sleep analysis can be found in rule-based and/or fuzzy systems for apneic event detection and hypnogram generation.[92–97] These systems implement explicit expert knowledge in the form of IF-THEN rules using linguistic terms. Although these *expert systems* are able to model general domain knowledge and enable traceability of the reasoning process, their design involves manual knowledge acquisition, feature engineering, and the establishment of a series of input and output space restrictions. This design is not scalable for modeling complex input–output relationships, unless design restrictions are relaxed and automatic parameterization by *learning from data* is implemented.[41,98] The procedure, however, is at the cost of significantly increasing the number and complexity of the associated internal rules, which are no longer fully expressed in interpretable linguistic terms. Similarly, machine-learning approaches that rely on handcrafted or normative features inherently constrain the degrees of freedom of the system because they have to deal with potentially suboptimal representations. At the other extreme one finds data-intensive DL approaches, which are very powerful for modeling large amounts of complex data but are often regarded as "black-boxes."[99]

The above stated trade-off does not mean that the possibility of finding a reasonable balance must be discarded.[100] Automatic PSG scoring can certainly benefit from future research in the area of explainable AI.[101] The recently introduced self-attention-based neural network architectures, for example, offer powerful prediction capabilities while providing user attention feedback. Recent applications of this technology have been proposed for sleep staging[14] and sleep apnea detection.[102] Transformer-based architectures, in addition, can overcome certain limitations of recurrent neural-network-based architectures in the analysis of longer data sequences.[103] Visualization feedback based on layer-wise relevance propagation networks has also been recently discussed in the context of automatic sleep staging.[72] Another promising approach is prototype learning, which combines DL with expert knowledge.[104] Areas of automatic PSG analysis other than sleep staging also stand to benefit from advances in this growing research field.

Another important aspect related to *trustfulness* is evaluation transparency and replicability. It is essential to have a common reference framework with which automatic scoring performance can be openly evaluated. This framework should include sufficiently large and representative open-access datasets with wide acceptance among sleep laboratories and scoring experts.[3] Ideally, access to the software or its source code should be granted. Finally, performance assessment methods and related terminology should be standardized to enable objective evaluations and comparisons in the context of common metrics and methodology.[105]

PRODUCTION DEPLOYMENT, USABILITY, DATA-PRIVACY, AND ETHICAL CONSIDERATIONS

The cost of transitioning from the controlled experimental conditions to the production environment can easily be underestimated. Most of the discussion in the preceding sections focused on the difficulties associated with the development and evaluation of automatic PSG analysis systems. The scalability of these systems, however, can also be compromised by more practical matters,

such as inadequate integration into practical end-user interfaces.[106–108] Clinicians must interact with software applications that offer efficient signal visualization and data analysis, a choice of scoring modalities, including manual scoring, and mechanisms for quality control and verification of outputs from full automatic analysis.[88,90]

Scoring software should be integrated into larger applications enabling efficient patient management and traceability of the clinical workflow. Interoperability with preexisting in-hospital or ambulatory technical infrastructure, such as hospital information systems and electronic health records, is essential. Software must also comply with data and medical device regulations, such as in Europe the General Data Protection Regulation[109] and the Medical Device Regulation.[110]

Efforts devoted to the accomplishment of these duties are considerably greater than those involved in developing the scoring algorithm itself. This is a task that mostly involves commercial companies with sufficient resources to adapt their products to meet the local specifications. Those companies would also manufacture and commercialize the fundamental pieces of hardware for patient monitoring and signal acquisition. Although hardware development is out of the scope of this study, the task entails notable challenges that need to be addressed. From a software standpoint, one obvious challenge regards smooth interfacing with these devices. In particular, scalable automatic analysis solutions should face the reality of a diversified and dynamic market with a variety of hardware specifications.

Cloud-based automatic PSG scoring can optimize resource use and facilitate hardware and software decoupling for analytical purposes. The centralization of computational resources for data-intensive methods such as DL is an interesting option for small, or non-IT-intensive, organizations. Examples of sleep systems in this category are Somnolyzer 24 × 7,[35,85] Z3Score,[111] EnsoSleep,[112] and Cerebra (previously Michelle)[113] sleep systems. This option, nevertheless, requires dealing with heterogeneous and proprietary data formats from different vendors across the client organizations. Reformatting data using open data formats, such as European Data Format (EDF+), can help the purpose.[114] Preadoption by the local entities of such standards as the default data storage option can facilitate matters even further and help (re)gain control of their data. A recurring question across hospital IT departments is as follows: "How are we going to keep all existing data in proprietary format, available and accessible, now that we want to switch provider?" Additional challenges for scalable cloud-based analysis solutions lie in the availability of secure, efficient network communication services. Specific data-privacy regulations also apply to the exchange, and possible out-of-clinic storage, of sensitive medical information.[115]

Considerations regarding preservation of data privacy, in fact, extend beyond operability in the production environment. The matter affects the development phase as well, particularly when building algorithms using data from multiple datasets (see "Interdatabase generalization and domain adaptation" section). Federated learning emerges as an interesting framework for overcoming limitations in this area. It eliminates the need for sensitive data sharing while enabling collaborative learning among a group of decentralized client nodes.[116] In the scope of federated learning, each dataset remains local at the owning node, whereas the learning process only involves exchanging of model parameters and aggregated descriptors. No information is leaked from the underlying data samples. Federated and self-supervised learning were recently applied to sleep staging for learning from diverse, unlabeled, private sensory data.[117]

As a final remark, the use of automatic PSG scoring, and more generally, AI-driven analysis in the medical domain, raises a number of ethical questions that need as well to be considered. Automatic learning from datasets, for example, can further exacerbate health inequities contained in data, such as racial, sex, or gender disparities.[118] These risks highlight the importance of clinicians retaining control of the process and the final diagnosis. Algorithm-based scoring outputs of the PSG must always be reviewed and, where necessary, rescored manually to ensure an accurate diagnosis and optimal patient care.[119]

BEYOND TRADITIONAL SLEEP SCORING: WHAT LIES AHEAD?

Future applications of AI in sleep medicine are expected to transcend current practices in PSG scoring.[119] The limitations of visual scoring have been highlighted on numerous occasions. Common concerns regard the assessment of sleep as a discontinuous process, artificial discretization on the basis of 30s analysis epochs, incomplete quantification of EEG and motor activity, or the use of ad hoc thresholds and definitions, sometimes merely conventional, or consensus-based, rather than extrapolated from data or physiological evidence.[120–123]

Sleep laboratories around the world collect vast amounts of mostly underused physiological data. Hours of physiological signals are reduced to summary metrics and indices that, at times, fail to correlate with meaningful diagnostic outcomes.[124] As an example, the diagnosis and treatment of obstructive sleep apnea has mostly been driven by the computation of one single metric, the so-called apnea-hypopnea index, whose limitations have been noted.[125,126]

Alternatively, computational methods have been developed that make use of novel physiological metrics that can be automatically extracted from the PSG. Together with the integration of –omics data, the new derived tools are expected to aid in the shift toward precision medicine.[37] Additional possibilities under investigation include personalized automatic sleep staging[71,72] and improved monitoring of the long-term health trajectories.[127]

The use of computer analysis for more continuous, probabilistic-based sleep state classification, which was proposed in the past,[97,120,128] has recently been revisited as *hypnodensity graph*[36,63] in the context of DL. This representation has shown its ability in modeling sleep staging ambiguity across several experts, achieving excellent reliability when compared with the classic consensus hypnogram. Moreover, it can provide a better framework for characterizing uncertainty underlying current methods of sleep stage classification.[24] Alike representations may have similar applications in the context of other areas related to PSG scoring.

In addition to already discussed applications of supervised ML, the use of this technique has been recently proposed for automatic detection of microsleep episodes[129] and improved characterization of sleep movement disorders.[84,130] Supervised ML, however, critically depends on the number and quality of examples contained in the learning dataset. It is also constrained by the specific configuration of the related input and output spaces. In other words, it cannot identify potentially novel categories or alternative characterizations of the discourse universe.[16,37] The possibilities of self-supervised, semisupervised, or unsupervised learning variants are exciting.[131] Unsupervised clustering, for example, has been used to identify obstructive sleep apnea subgroups and phenotypes missed by conventional classification systems.[132] It may be that the higher interrater variability rates observed for the scoring of stage N1 are explained by the existence of additional subphases yet to be discovered.[16] Unsupervised and data-driven approaches have been proposed in this line for capturing unknown distinctive features or latent states.[133–135]

AI-driven technology for the analysis of physiological activity recorded by wearable devices deserves special mention.[136] Sleep tracking apps have gained popularity among the general population due to their affordability, ease-of-use, and ubiquity. These characteristics make them attractive candidates for enabling long-term out-of-clinic monitoring and new screening possibilities.[137] An in-depth discussion on the specifics of these devices would exceed the scope of this article but the interested reader is referred to several recent approaches[49,73,138–141] and 2 reviews providing a more systematic analysis of the sensing technologies and analytical methods involved.[142,143]

The disruptive eruption of these devices in the consumer market, however, poses a series of challenges, both from the clinical and the user perspective. The technology provides an excellent opportunity to promote participatory medicine by fostering people to be active agents in their health management.[144] However, taking that too far can lead to excessive concern about reaching "normative sleep."[145] The integration of wearable health technology into clinical settings must be carefully deliberated, with attention paid to issues such as electronic health record integration, billing, and quality metrics.[146,147] Perhaps more importantly, despite its market penetration, consumer sleep tracking technology remains largely unregulated.[142,148] The lack of access to the raw data and algorithms used by some of the commercial systems available may raise doubts about the reliability of these systems and their usefulness for clinical and research purposes.[149] The more challenging monitoring conditions in comparison to attended in-laboratory PSG (eg, limited sensing, changing environment, or broader presence of intersubject differences) would inevitably compromise the quality and the information content of the associated physiological signals collected by these devices.

Scientific societies have a fundamental role to play in the standardization of related terminology and performance assessment procedures. A number of guidelines already exist, such as those proposed by the American Academy of Sleep Medicine (AASM) Consumer and Clinical Technology Committee[150] or the joint initiative of the Consumer Technology Association and the National Sleep Foundation.[151–153] Independent research groups have also developed best practices for validation studies and guidelines on how to choose a wearable device for research and clinical use.[154] These recommendations led to a recent proposal for a standardized framework with step-by-step guidelines and open-source code for performance evaluation of consumer sleep technology.[155] Another recent study with a broader scope published guidelines for reporting rigorous performance evaluation of novel sleep health technologies.[105]

In conclusion, although challenges remain to be solved for effective large-scale deployment of automatic PSG scoring, recent technology developments are rapidly closing the gap. An exciting near future lies ahead for researchers, clinicians, and companies involved in the inmediate development of this field.

CLINICS CARE POINTS

- Computer-assisted polysomnography analysis can significantly lower down the costs and improve consistency of the test results associated to the diagnosis of sleep disorders.
- Patients can benefit from shortened waiting lists resulting from the more efficient sleep clinic workflow.
- A number of relevant topics remain open on the research plane, but the basic technology is ready.
- Automatic analysis has to be implemented into usable software tools that integrate with the existing technical and clinical infrastructure.
- Special attention should be focused toward key aspects in the resulting decision-making regarding human agency and oversight, patient safety, technical robustness, data-privacy, transparency, fairness, and accountability.
- Close collaboration between manufacturers, policy makers, and on-site technical and clinical staff is needed for achieving this goal in compliance with evolving regulation.

DISCLOSURE

No conflicts of interest to declare.

ACKNOWLEDGMENTS

The author wants to thank funding received under project ED431H 2020/10 of Xunta de Galicia, and the support from the Centro de Investigación de Galicia, Spain (CITIC), funded by Xunta de Galicia through a collaboration agreement between the Regional Ministry of Culture, Education, and Vocational Training and the Galician Universities for the work of the Research Centers of the Galician University System and the Handytronic chair.

REFERENCES

1. Berry R., Brooks R., Gamaldo C., et al., The AASM manual for the scoring of sleep and associated events: rules, terminology and technical specifications, version 2.6, 2020, American Academy of Sleep Medicine; Darien, IL.

2. Younes M, Raneri J, Hanly P. Staging sleep in polysomnograms: analysis of inter-scorer variability. J Clin Sleep Med 2016;12(06):885–94.

3. Penzel T. Sleep scoring moving from visual scoring towards automated scoring. Sleep 2022. https://doi.org/10.1093/sleep/zsac190. zsac190.

4. Lee YJ, Lee JY, Cho JH, et al. Interrater reliability of sleep stage scoring: a meta-analysis. J Clin Sleep Med 2022;18(1):193–202.

5. Smith JR, Negin M, Nevis AH. Automatic analysis of sleep electroencephalograms by hybrid computation. IEEE Trans Syst Sci Cybern 1969;5(4):278–84.

6. Gaillard JM, Simmen AE, Tissot R. Analyse automatique des enregistrements polygraphiques de sommeil. Electroencephalogr Clin Neurophysiol 1971;30(6):557–61.

7. Penzel T, Conradt R. Computer based sleep recording and analysis. Sleep Med Rev 2000;4(2):131–48.

8. Alvarez-Estevez D, Morel-Bonillo V. Computer-assisted diagnosis of the sleep apnea-hypopnea syndrome: a review. Sleep Disord 2015;2015:1–33.

9. Fiorillo L, Puiatti A, Papandrea M, et al. Automated sleep scoring: a review of the latest approaches. Sleep Med Rev 2019;48:101204.

10. Mostafa SS, Mendonca F, Ravelo-García A G. A systematic review of detecting sleep apnea using deep learning. Sensors 2019;19(22):4934.

11. Qian X, Qiu Y, He Q, et al. A review of methods for sleep arousal detection using polysomnographic signals. Brain Sci 2021;11(10):1274.

12. Younes M. The case for using digital EEG analysis in clinical sleep medicine. Sleep Sci Pract 2017;1(1):2.

13. Russell SJ, Norvig P. Artificial intelligence: a modern approach. 4th edition, global edition. Hoboken, NJ: Pearson; 2022.

14. Phan H, Mikkelsen K, Chen OY, et al. SleepTransformer: automatic sleep staging with interpretability and uncertainty quantification. IEEE Trans Biomed Eng 2022;69(8):2456–67.

15. Gutiérrez-Tobal GC, Álvarez D, Vaquerizo-Villar F, Penzel T, Hornero R, et al. Advances in the Diagnosis and Treatment of sleep apnea. Vol 1384. In: Advances in experimental medicine and Biology. Cham, Switzerland: Springer Nature Switzerland AG; 2022. p. 131–46.

16. de Chazal P, Mazzotti DR, Cistulli PA. Automated sleep staging algorithms: have we reached the performance limit due to manual scoring? Sleep 2022;1–3. https://doi.org/10.1093/sleep/zsac159.

17. Whitney C, Gottlieb D, Redline S, et al. Reliability of scoring respiratory disturbance indices and sleep staging. Sleep 1998;21:749–57.

18. Ferri R, Ferri P, Colognola R, et al. Comparison between the results of an automatic and a visual scoring of sleep EEG recordings. Sleep 1989. https://doi.org/10.1093/sleep/12.4.354.

19. Norman R, Pal I, Stewart C, et al. Interobserver agreement among sleep scorers from different centers in a large dataset. Sleep 2000;23:901–8.

20. Collop NA. Scoring variability between polysomnography technologists in different sleep laboratories. Sleep Med 2002;3(1):43–7.

21. Malhotra A, Younes M, Kuna ST, et al. Performance of an automated polysomnography scoring system versus computer-assisted manual scoring. Sleep 2013;36(4):573–82.

22. Berthomier C, Muto V, Schmidt C, et al. Exploring scoring methods for research studies: accuracy and variability of visual and automated sleep scoring. J Sleep Res 2020;29(5). https://doi.org/10.1111/jsr.12994.

23. Alvarez-Estevez D, Rijsman RM. Inter-database validation of a deep learning approach for automatic sleep scoring. PLoS One 2021;16:e0256111. Qiu Y.

24. Bakker JP, Ross M, Cerny A, et al. Scoring sleep with artificial intelligence enables quantification of sleep stage ambiguity: hypnodensity based on multiple expert scorers and auto-scoring. Sleep 2022;zsac154. https://doi.org/10.1093/sleep/zsac154.

25. Magalang UJ, Chen NH, Cistulli PA, et al. Agreement in the scoring of respiratory events and sleep among international sleep centers. Sleep 2013;36(4):591–6.

26. Kuna ST, Benca R, Kushida CA, et al. Agreement in computer-assisted manual scoring of polysomnograms across sleep centers. Sleep 2013;36(4):583–9.

27. Alvarez-Estevez D, Rijsman RM. Computer-assisted analysis of polysomnographic recordings improves inter-scorer associated agreement and scoring times. PLoS One 2022;17:e0275530. Veauthier C.

28. Alvarez-Estevez D, Fernández-Varela I. Addressing database variability in learning from medical data: an ensemble-based approach using convolutional neural networks and a case of study applied to automatic sleep scoring. Comput Biol Med 2020;119:103697.

29. Ferri R, Fulda S, Allen RP, et al. World Association of Sleep Medicine (WASM) 2016 standards for recording and scoring leg movements in polysomnograms developed by a joint task force from the

International and the European Restless Legs Syndrome Study Groups (IRLSSG and EURLSSG). Sleep Med 2016;26:86–95.

30. Danker-Hopfe H, Anderer P, Zeitlhofer J, et al. Inter-rater reliability for sleep scoring according to the Rechtschaffen & Kales and the new AASM standard. J Sleep Res 2009;18:74–84.

31. Rosenberg R, van Hout S. The American Academy of Sleep Medicine inter-scorer reliability program: sleep stage scoring. J Clin Sleep Med 2013;9:81–7.

32. Magalang UJ, Arnardottir ES, Chen NH, et al. Agreement in the scoring of respiratory events among international sleep centers for home sleep testing. J Clin Sleep Med 2016;12(01):71–7.

33. van Gorp H, Huijben IAM, Fonseca P, et al. Certainty about uncertainty in sleep staging: a theoretical framework. Sleep 2022;45(8):zsac134.

34. Padovano D, Martinez-Rodrigo A, Pastor JM, et al. On the generalization of sleep apnea detection methods based on heart rate variability and machine learning. IEEE Access 2022;10:92710–25.

35. Punjabi NM, Shifa N, Dorffner G, et al. Computer-assisted automated scoring of polysomnograms using the somnolyzer system. Sleep 2015;38(10): 1555–66.

36. Stephansen J, Olesen A, Olsen M, et al. Neural network analysis of sleep stages enables efficient diagnosis of narcolepsy. Nat Commun 2018;9: 1–15.

37. Lim DC, Mazzotti DR, Sutherland K, et al. Reinventing polysomnography in the age of precision medicine. Sleep Med Rev 2020;52:101313.

38. Goldberger AL, Amaral LAN, Glass L, et al. Components of a new research resource for complex physiologic signals. Circulation 2000;101(23). https://doi.org/10.1161/01.CIR.101.23.e215.

39. Zhang GQ, Cui L, Mueller R, et al. The national sleep research resource: towards a sleep data commons. J Am Med Inform Assoc 2018;25(10): 1351–8.

40. Fulda S. Periodic leg movements during sleep. Sleep Med Clin 2021;16(2):289–303.

41. Bishop CM. Pattern recognition and machine learning. New York, NY: Springer; 2006.

42. Tsinalis O, Matthews P, Guo Y. Automatic sleep stage scoring using time-frequency analysis and stacked sparse autoencoders. Ann Biomed Eng 2016;44:1587–97.

43. Olsen M, Schneider LD, Cheung J, et al. Automatic, electrocardiographic-based detection of autonomic arousals and their association with cortical arousals, leg movements, and respiratory events in sleep. Sleep 2018;41(3). https://doi.org/10.1093/sleep/zsy006.

44. Sun H, Jia J, Goparaju B, et al. Large-scale automated sleep staging. Sleep 2017;40(10). https://doi.org/10.1093/sleep/zsx139.

45. Phan H, Andreotti F, Cooray N, et al. SeqSleepNet: end-to-end hierarchical recurrent neural network for sequence-to-sequence automatic sleep staging. IEEE Trans Neural Syst Rehabil Eng 2019; 27(3):400–10.

46. Mousavi S, Afghah F, Acharya UR. SleepEEGNet: automated sleep stage scoring with sequence to sequence deep learning approach. In: Pławiak P, editor. PLoS One 2019;14(5):e0216456.

47. Erdenebayar U, Kim YJ, Park JU, et al. Deep learning approaches for automatic detection of sleep apnea events from an electrocardiogram. Comput Methods Programs Biomed 2019;180: 105001.

48. Nikkonen S, Korkalainen H, Leino A, et al. Automatic respiratory event scoring in obstructive sleep apnea using a long short-term memory neural network. IEEE J Biomed Health Inform 2021; 25(8):2917–27.

49. Wulterkens BM, Fonseca P, Hermans LW, et al. It is all in the wrist: wearable sleep staging in a clinical population versus reference polysomnography. Nat Sci Sleep 2021;13:885–97.

50. Casal R, Di Persia LE, Schlotthauer G. Temporal convolutional networks and transformers for classifying the sleep stage in awake or asleep using pulse oximetry signals. J Comput Sci 2022;59: 101544.

51. Lin YS, Wu YP, Wu YC, et al. Achieving accurate automatic sleep apnea/hypopnea syndrome assessment using nasal pressure signal. IEEE J Biomed Health Inform 2022;1–10. https://doi.org/10.1109/JBHI.2022.3199454.

52. Hassan AR, Bhuiyan MIH. A decision support system for automatic sleep staging from EEG signals using tunable Q-factor wavelet transform and spectral features. J Neurosci Methods 2016;271: 107–18.

53. Supratak A, Dong H, Wu C, et al. DeepSleepNet: a model for automatic sleep stage scoring based on raw single-channel EEG. IEEE Trans Neural Netw Rehabil Eng 2017;25:1998–2008.

54. Brink-Kjaer A, Olesen AN, Peppard PE, et al. Automatic detection of cortical arousals in sleep and their contribution to daytime sleepiness. Clin Neurophysiol 2020;131(6):1187–203.

55. Eldele E, Chen Z, Liu C, et al. An attention-based deep learning approach for sleep stage classification with single-channel EEG. IEEE Trans Neural Syst Rehabil Eng 2021;29:809–18.

56. Li H, Guan Y. DeepSleep convolutional neural network allows accurate and fast detection of sleep arousal. Commun Biol 2021;4(1):18.

57. Bresch E, Großekathöfer U, Garcia-Molina G. Recurrent deep neural networks for real-time sleep stage classification from single channel EEG. Front Comput Neurosci 2018;12:85.

58. Malafeev A, Laptev D, Bauer S, et al. Automatic human sleep stage scoring using deep neural networks. Front Neurosci 2018;12:781.

59. Biswal S, Sun H, Goparaju B, et al. Expert-level sleep scoring with deep neural networks. J Am Med Inform Assoc 2018;25(12):1643–50.

60. Zhang L, Fabbri D, Upender R, et al. Automated sleep stage scoring of the Sleep Heart Health Study using deep neural networks. Sleep 2019; 42(11):zsz159.

61. Li A, Chen S, Quan SF, et al. A deep learning-based algorithm for detection of cortical arousal during sleep. Sleep 2020;43(12):10.

62. Olesen AN, Jørgen Jennum P, Mignot E, et al. Automatic sleep stage classification with deep residual networks in a mixed-cohort setting. Sleep 2021; 44(1):zsaa161.

63. Cesari M, Stefani A, Penzel T, et al. Interrater sleep stage scoring reliability between manual scoring from two European sleep centers and automatic scoring performed by the artificial intelligence–based Stanford-STAGES algorithm. J Clin Sleep Med 2021;17(6):1237–47.

64. Qin H, Liu G. A dual-model deep learning method for sleep apnea detection based on representation learning and temporal dependence. Neurocomputing 2022;473:24–36.

65. Perslev M, Darkner S, Kempfner L, et al. U-Sleep: resilient high-frequency sleep staging. Npj Digit Med 2021;4(1):72.

66. Guillot A, Thorey V. RobustSleepNet: transfer learning for automated sleep staging at scale. IEEE Trans Neural Syst Rehabil Eng 2021;29:1441–51.

67. Fiorillo L, Pedroncelli D, Agostini V, et al. Multi-scored sleep databases: how to exploit the multiple-labels in automated sleep scoring. arxiv 2022. https://doi.org/10.48550/ARXIV.2207.01910.

68. Pan SJ, Yang Q. A survey on transfer learning. IEEE Trans Knowl Data Eng 2010;22(10):1345–59.

69. Chambon S, Galtier MN, Gramfort A. Domain adaptation with optimal transport improves EEG sleep stage classifiers. International workshop on pattern recognition in neuroimaging (PRNI), IEEE 2018;1–4.

70. Abou Jaoude M, Sun H, Pellerin KR, et al. Expert-level automated sleep staging of long-term scalp electroencephalography recordings using deep learning. Sleep 2020;43(11):zsaa112.

71. Phan H, Mikkelsen K, Chén OY, et al. Personalized automatic sleep staging with single-night data: a pilot study with Kullback–Leibler divergence regularization. Physiol Meas 2020;41(6):064004.

72. Banluesombatkul N, Ouppaphan P, Leelaarporn P, et al. MetaSleepLearner: a pilot study on fast adaptation of bio-signals-based sleep stage classifier to new individual subject using meta-learning. IEEE J Biomed Health Inform 2021;25(6):1949–63.

73. Radha M, Fonseca P, Moreau A, et al. A deep transfer learning approach for wearable sleep stage classification with photoplethysmography. Npj Digit Med 2021;4(1):135.

74. Phan H, Chen OY, Koch P, et al. Towards more accurate automatic sleep staging via deep transfer learning. IEEE Trans Biomed Eng 2021;68(6): 1787–98.

75. Eldele E, Ragab M, Chen Z, et al. ADAST: attentive cross-domain EEG-based sleep staging framework with iterative self-training. IEEE Trans Emerg Top Comput Intell 2022;1–12. https://doi.org/10.1109/TETCI.2022.3189695.

76. Zhao R, Xia Y, Zhang Y. Unsupervised sleep staging system based on domain adaptation. Biomed Signal Process Control 2021;69:102937.

77. Yoo C, Lee HW, Kang JW. Transferring structured knowledge in unsupervised domain adaptation of a sleep staging network. IEEE J Biomed Health Inform 2022;26(3):1273–84.

78. Fan J, Zhu H, Jiang X, et al. Unsupervised domain adaptation by statistics alignment for deep sleep staging networks. IEEE Trans Neural Syst Rehabil Eng 2022;30:205–16.

79. Nasiri S., Clifford G.D., Attentive adversarial network for large-scale sleep staging. In: Doshi-Velez F., Fackler J., Jung K., et al., eds. Proceedings of the 5th machine Learning for healthcare conference. Vol 126. Proceedings of machine learning research PMLR; 2020:457-478. Available at: https://proceedings.mlr.press/v126/nasiri20a.html. Accessed October 24, 2022.

80. Phan H, Mikkelsen K. Automatic sleep staging of EEG signals: recent development, challenges, and future directions. Physiol Meas 2022;43(4): 04TR01.

81. Pittman S, MacDonald M, Fogel R, et al. Assessment of automated scoring of polysomnographic recordings in a population with suspected sleep-disordered breathing. Sleep 2004;27:1394–403.

82. Younes M, Younes M, Giannouli E. Accuracy of automatic polysomnography scoring using frontal electrodes. J Clin Sleep Med 2016;12(05):735–46.

83. Guillot A, Sauvet F, During EH, et al. Dreem open datasets: multi-scored sleep datasets to compare human and automated sleep staging. IEEE Trans Neural Syst Rehabil Eng 2020;28(9):1955–65.

84. Carvelli L, Olesen AN, Brink-Kjaer A, et al. Design of a deep learning model for automatic scoring of periodic and non-periodic leg movements during sleep validated against multiple human experts. Sleep Med 2020;69:109–19.

85. Anderer P, Moreau A, Woertz M, et al. Computer-assisted sleep classification according to the standard of the American academy of sleep medicine: validation study of the AASM version of the somnolyzer 24 × 7. Neuropsychobiology 2010;62(4):250–64.

86. Koupparis AM, Kokkinos V, Kostopoulos GK. Semi-automatic sleep EEG scoring based on the hypnospectrogram. J Neurosci Methods 2014;221: 189–95.

87. Svetnik V, Ma J, Soper KA, et al. Evaluation of automated and semi-automated scoring of polysomnographic recordings from a clinical trial using zolpidem in the treatment of insomnia. Sleep 2007;30(11):1562–74.

88. Younes M, Hanly PJ. Minimizing interrater variability in staging sleep by use of computer-derived features. J Clin Sleep Med 2016;12(10): 1347–56.

89. Younes M, Thompson W, Leslie C, et al. Utility of technologist editing of polysomnography scoring performed by a validated automatic system. Ann Am Thorac Soc 2015. https://doi.org/10.1513/AnnalsATS.201411-512OC. 150611180544002.

90. Anderer P, Gruber G, Parapatics S, et al. An E-health solution for automatic sleep classification according to rechtschaffen and kales: validation study of the somnolyzer 24 × 7 utilizing the siesta database. Neuropsychobiology 2005;51(3):115–33.

91. Linardatos P, Papastefanopoulos V, Kotsiantis S. Explainable AI: a review of machine learning interpretability methods. Entropy 2020;23(1):18.

92. Daniels JE, Cayton RM, Chappell MJ, et al. Cadosa: a fuzzy expert system for differential diagnosis of obstructive sleep apnoea and related conditions. Expert Syst Appl 1997;12(2):163–77.

93. Fred A, Filipe J, Partinen M, et al. An expert system for the diagnosis of sleep disorders. Stud Health Technol Inf 2000;78:127–47.

94. Otero A. Algorithms for the analysis of polysomnographic recordings with customizable criteria. Expert Syst Appl 2011;14:10133–46.

95. Cabrero-Canosa M, Castro-Pereiro M, Grana-Ramos M, et al. An intelligent system for the detection and interpretation of sleep apneas. Expert Syst Appl 2003;15:335–49.

96. Álvarez-Estévez D, Moret-Bonillo V. Fuzzy reasoning used to detect apneic events in the sleep apnea-hypopnea syndrome. Expert Syst Appl 2009;36(4): 7778–85.

97. Alvarez-Estevez D, Fernandez-Pastoriza J, Hernandez-Pereira E, et al. A method for the automatic analysis of the sleep macrostructure in continuum. Expert Syst Appl 2013;40:1796–803.

98. Jang JSR. ANFIS: adaptive-network-based fuzzy inference system. IEEE Trans Syst Man Cybern 1993;23(3):665–85.

99. Goodfellow I., Bengio Y. and Courville A., Deep learning, 2016, MIT Press, Cambridge, MA.

100. Alonso Moral JM, Castiello C, Magdalena L, et al. Explainable fuzzy systems: paving the way from interpretable fuzzy systems to explainable AI systems. Springer Nature Switzerland AG, Cham, Switzerland; 2021.

101. Arrieta AB. Explainable Artificial Intelligence (XAI): concepts, taxonomies, opportunities and challenges toward responsible AI. Inf Fusion 2020;34.

102. Hu S, Cai W, Gao T, et al. A hybrid transformer model for obstructive sleep apnea detection based on self-attention mechanism using single-lead ECG. IEEE Trans Instrum Meas 2022;71:1–11.

103. Vaswani A, Shazeer N, Parmar N, et al. Attention Is All You Need. 2017. Available at: http://arxiv.org/abs/1706.03762. Accessed September 19, 2022.

104. Al-Hussaini I, Xiao C, Westover MB, et al. SLEEPER: interpretable sleep staging via prototypes from expert rules. In: Doshi-Velez F, Fackler J, Jung K, et al., eds. Proceedings of the 4th machine learning for healthcare conference. Vol 106. Proceedings of machine learning research. PMLR; 2019:721-739. Available at: https://proceedings.mlr.press/v106/al-hussaini19a.html.

105. de Zambotti M, Menghini L, Grandner MA, et al. Rigorous performance evaluation (previously, "validation") for informed use of new technologies for sleep health measurement. Sleep Health 2022; 8(3):263–9.

106. Alonso-Ríos D, Vázquez-García A, Mosqueira-Rey E, et al. A critical analysis and a taxonomy. Int J Hum-Comput Interact 2009;26(1):53–74.

107. Marcilly R, Peute L, Beuscart-Zephir MC. From usability engineering to evidence-based usability in health IT. Stud Health Technol Inf 2016;222:126–38.

108. Carayon P, Hoonakker P. Human factors and usability for health information technology: old and new challenges. Yearb Med Inform 2019;28(01): 071–7.

109. European Commission. Regulation (EU) 2016/679 of the European Parliament and of the Council of 27 April 2016 on the protection of natural persons with regard to the processing of personal data and on the free movement of such data, and repealing Directive 95/46/EC (General Data Protection Regulation) (Text with EEA relevance). Published online 2016. Available at: https://eur-lex.europa.eu/eli/reg/2016/679/oj. Accessed October 24, 2022.

110. European Commission. Regulation (EU) 2017/745 of the European Parliament and of the Council of 5 April 2017 on medical devices, amending Directive 2001/83/EC, Regulation (EC) No 178/2002 and Regulation (EC) No 1223/2009 and repealing Council Directives 90/385/EEC and 93/42/EEC (Text with EEA relevance). Published online 2017. Available at: http://data.europa.eu/eli/reg/2017/745/oj. Accessed October 24, 2022.

111. Z3Score - Cloud AI powered automatic sleep scoring system Available at: https://z3score.com/. Accessed October 24, 2022.

112. Home. EnsoData Available at: https://www. ensodata.com/. Accessed October 24, 2022.

113. Cerebra - Putting the Sleep Back Into Sleep Medicine. Cerebra. Available at: https://www.cerebra. health/. Accessed October 24, 2022.

114. Kemp B, Olivan J. European data format "plus" (EDF+), an EDF alike standard format for the exchange of physiological data. Clin Neurophysiol 2003;114:1755–61.

115. Ali O, Shrestha A, Soar J, et al. Cloud computing-enabled healthcare opportunities, issues, and applications: a systematic review. Int J Inf Manag 2018;43:146–58.

116. Yang Q., Liu Y., Chen T., Tong Y., Federated Machine Learning: Concept and Applications. Published online February 13, 2019. Accessed October 24, 2022. Available at: http://arxiv.org/abs/1902.04885. Accessed October 24, 2022.

117. Saeed A, Salim FD, Ozcelebi T, et al. Federated self-supervised learning of multisensor representations for embedded intelligence. IEEE Internet Things J 2021;8(2):1030–40.

118. Chen IY, Pierson E, Rose S, et al. Ethical machine learning in healthcare. Annu Rev Biomed Data Sci 2021;4(1):123–44.

119. Goldstein CA, Berry RB, Kent DT, et al. Artificial intelligence in sleep medicine: an American Academy of Sleep Medicine position statement. J Clin Sleep Med 2020;16(4):3.

120. Pardey J, Roberts S, Tarassenko L, et al. A new approach to the analysis of the human sleep/wakefulness continuum. J Sleep Res 1996;5(4):201–10.

121. Himanen SL, Hasan J, Limitations of Rechtschaffen and Kales. Sleep Med Rev 2000;4(2):149–67.

122. Schulz H. Rethinking sleep analysis: comment on the AASM manual for the scoring of sleep and associated events. J Clin Sleep Med 2008;04(02): 99–103.

123. Parrino L, Ferri R, Zucconi M, et al. Commentary from the Italian Association of Sleep Medicine on the AASM manual for the scoring of sleep and associated events: for debate and discussion. Sleep Med 2009;10(7):799–808.

124. Zinchuk A, Yaggi HK. Sleep apnea heterogeneity, phenotypes, and cardiovascular risk. Implications for trial design and precision sleep medicine. Am J Respir Crit Care Med 2019;200(4):412–3.

125. Borsini E, Nogueira F, Nigro C. Apnea-hypopnea index in sleep studies and the risk of over-simplification. Sleep Sci 2018;11(1):45–8.

126. Malhotra A, Ayappa I, Ayas N, et al. Metrics of sleep apnea severity: beyond the apnea-hypopnea index. Sleep 2021;44(7):zsab030.

127. Schmickl CN, Heckman E, Owens RL, et al. The respiratory signature: a novel concept to leverage continuous positive airway pressure therapy as an early warning system for exacerbations of common diseases such as heart failure. J Clin Sleep Med 2019;15(06):923–7.

128. Flexer A, Gruber G, Dorffner G. A reliable probabilistic sleep stager based on a single EEG signal. Artif Intell Med 2005;33(3):199–207.

129. Malafeev A, Hertig-Godeschalk A, Schreier DR, et al. Automatic detection of microsleep episodes with deep learning. Front Neurosci 2021;15:564098.

130. Cesari M, Christensen JAE, Muntean ML, et al. A data-driven system to identify REM sleep behavior disorder and to predict its progression from the prodromal stage in Parkinson's disease. Sleep Med 2021;77:238–48.

131. Jing L, Tian Y. Self-supervised visual feature learning with deep neural networks: a survey. IEEE Trans Pattern Anal Mach Intell 2021;43(11): 4037–58.

132. Zinchuk AV, Jeon S, Koo BB, et al. Polysomnographic phenotypes and their cardiovascular implications in obstructive sleep apnoea. Thorax 2018; 73(5):472–80.

133. Koch H, Christensen JAE, Frandsen R, et al. Automatic sleep classification using a data-driven topic model reveals latent sleep states. J Neurosci Methods 2014;235:130–7.

134. Stevner ABA, Vidaurre D, Cabral J, et al. Discovery of key whole-brain transitions and dynamics during human wakefulness and non-REM sleep. Nat Commun 2019;10(1):1035.

135. Decat N, Walter J, Koh ZH, et al. Beyond traditional sleep scoring: massive feature extraction and data driven clustering of sleep time series. Sleep Med 2022;98:39–52. https://doi.org/10.1016/j.sleep. 2022.06.013.

136. de Zambotti M, Menghini L, Cellini N, et al. Performance of consumer wearable sleep technology, Kushida C.A. In: Encyclopedia of Sleep and Circadian Rhythms. Second Edition. Academic Press; 2023. p. 6–15.

137. Tobin SY, Williams PG, Baron KG, et al. Challenges and opportunities for applying wearable technology to sleep. Sleep Med Clin 2021;16(4):607–18.

138. Korkalainen H, Aakko J, Duce B, et al. Deep learning enables sleep staging from photoplethysmogram for patients with suspected sleep apnea. Sleep 2020;43(11):zsaa098.

139. Olsen M, Zeitzer JM, Richardson RN, et al. A flexible deep learning architecture for temporal sleep stage classification using accelerometry and photoplethysmography. IEEE Trans Biomed Eng 2022;1–10. https://doi.org/10.1109/TBME. 2022.3187945.

140. Thiesse L, Staner L, Bourgin P, et al. Validation of Somno-Art Software, a novel approach of sleep staging, compared with polysomnography in disturbed sleep profiles. SLEEP Adv 2022;3(1): zpab019.

141. Thiesse L, Staner L, Fuchs G, et al. Performance of Somno-Art Software compared to polysomnography interscorer variability: a multi-center study. Sleep Med 2022;96:14–9.

142. de Zambotti M, Cellini N, Menghini L, et al. Sensors capabilities, performance, and use of consumer sleep technology. Sleep Med Clin 2020;15(1):1–30.

143. Imtiaz SA. A systematic review of sensing technologies for wearable sleep staging. Sensors 2021; 21(5):1562.

144. Nieto-Riveiro L, Groba B, Miranda MC, et al. Technologies for participatory medicine and health promotion in the elderly population. Medicine (Baltim) 2018;97(20):e10791.

145. Baron KG, Abbott S, Jao N, et al. Orthosomnia: are some patients taking the quantified self too far? J Clin Sleep Med 2017;13(02):351–4.

146. Khosla S, Deak MC, Gault D, et al. Consumer sleep technology: an American academy of sleep medicine position statement. J Clin Sleep Med 2018; 14(05):877–80.

147. Khosla S, Deak MC, Gault D, et al. Consumer sleep technologies: how to balance the promises of new technology with evidence-based medicine and clinical guidelines. J Clin Sleep Med 2019;15(01): 163–5.

148. Baumert M, Cowie MR, Redline S, et al. Sleep characterization with smart wearable devices: a call for standardization and consensus recommendations. Sleep 2022;zsac183. https://doi.org/10.1093/sleep/zsac183.

149. Ameen MS, Cheung LM, Hauser T. About the accuracy and problems of consumer devices in the assessment of sleep. Sensors 2019;19(19):4160.

150. Schutte-Rodin S, Deak MC, Khosla S, et al. Evaluating consumer and clinical sleep technologies: an American Academy of Sleep Medicine update. J Clin Sleep Med 2021;17(11):2275–82.

151. Consumer Technology Association. Definitions and Characteristics for Wearable Sleep Monitors (ANSI/CTA/NSF-2052.1-A). Published online 2022. Available at: https://shop.cta.tech/collections/standards/products/definitions-and-characteristics-for-wearable-sleep-monitors-ansi-cta-nsf-2052-1-a. Accessed October 24, 2022.

152. Consumer Technology Association. Methodology of Measurements for Features in Sleep Tracking Consumer Technology devices and Applications (ANSI/CTA/NSF- 2052.2). Published online 2017. Available at: https://shop.cta.tech/products/methodology-of-measurements-for-features-in-sleep-tracking-consumer-technology-devices-and-applications. Accessed October 24, 2022.

153. Consumer Technology Association. Performance Criteria and Testing Protocols for Features in Sleep Tracking Consumer Technology Devices and Applications (ANSI/CTA/NSF-2052.3). Published online 2019. Available at: https://shop.cta.tech/products/performance-criteria-and-testing-protocols-for-features-in-sleep-tracking-consumer-technology-devices-and-applications. Accessed October 24, 2022.

154. Depner CM, Cheng PC, Devine JK, et al. Wearable technologies for developing sleep and circadian biomarkers: a summary of workshop discussions. Sleep 2020;43(2):zsz254.

155. Menghini L, Cellini N, Goldstone A, et al. A standardized framework for testing the performance of sleep-tracking technology: step-by-step guidelines and open-source code. Sleep 2021; 44(2):zsaa170.

Unmasking Heterogeneity of Sleep Apnea

Allan I. Pack, MBChB, PhD

KEYWORDS

- Obstructive sleep apnea • Risk factors for OSA • Symptoms of OSA • Hypoxic burden
- Heart rate response to events

KEY POINTS

- Obstructive sleep apnea (OSA) is a very heterogeneous disorder in multiple dimensions.
- There are different physiological risk factors.
- There are different clinical subtypes of OSA.
- The preponderance of evidence indicates that the excessively sleepy subtype is at increased risk of future cardiovascular (CV) events if OSA is untreated.
- New metrics of the physiological derangements in OSA—hypoxic burden and heart rate response to events—may provide information on who with OSA is at most risk for cardiovascular consequences.

Obstructive sleep apnea (OSA) is a common disorder.[1] There is growing evidence that there is substantial heterogeneity among patients with the same apparent severity of disease. There are multiple dimensions to this heterogeneity. This includes the following: (1) physiological risk factors for the disorder, (2) symptom subtypes, and (3) physiological consequences of the breathing disorder during sleep. In this brief review, we will discuss each of these aspects.

PHYSIOLOGICAL RISK FACTORS FOR OBSTRUCTIVE SLEEP APNEA

It has been proposed that there are 4 major physiological risk factors for OSA, that is, (1) airway collapsibility, (2) overall loop gain–a measure of stability of the ventilatory control system, (3) arousal threshold, and (d) muscle responsiveness, that is, the increase in activity of upper airway dilator muscles because of the reflex driven by negative intraluminal pressure.[2] Early studies sought to estimate these different risk factors using a complex laboratory protocol that involved recording of activity of a representative upper airway dilator muscle, that is, genioglossus, as

well as intraluminal pressure in the upper airway.[3] The protocol to do this was complex and, while of research value, was not clinically applicable.

More recently there have been efforts to determine these 4 variables from the assessment of data collected during routine polysomnography. This is based on a simple model of ventilatory control.[4] The concept is that one seeks to match the model output with the measured nasal pressure during sleep. This approach is controversial. Younes and Schwab have indicated that the very simple model that is the basis of this approach is based on untenable assumptions.[5] The key assumptions they challenged are the following: (1) that following an arousal and resumption of ventilation at the end of an obstructive event the airway is always completely open and (2) that the effect of arousal is the same for all events within an individual. There are different intensities of arousal[6] that are not accounted for. Proponents of this approach accept these are reasonable concerns as stated in a Pro-Con debate.[7]

Currently, we do not know how big an effect these concerns have on the results obtained, and this has not been assessed in sensitivity analyses. There are additional concerns about this approach

Division of Sleep Medicine, Department of Medicine, University of Pennsylvania, Perelman School of Medicine, 125 South 31st Street, Translational Reseasrch Laboratories, Suite 2100, Philadelphia, PA 19104, USA
E-mail address: pack@pennmedicine.upenn.edu

Sleep Med Clin 18 (2023) 293–299
https://doi.org/10.1016/j.jsmc.2023.05.003
1556-407X/23/© 2023 Elsevier Inc. All rights reserved.

sleep.theclinics.com

because data on independent validation of the measures obtained are rather sparse and recent data on night-to-night agreement of the results obtained are not that encouraging.[8,9]

Despite the lack of these important data, there has been a relatively large number of articles published using this approach. Differences between physiological risk factors in men and women have been described.[10] The approach has also been used to provide information of potential clinical value, that is, to determine these subtypes of patients with OSA who will respond to intraoral devices and those who will not.[11,12]

Although of some interest, these results need to be considered as tentative because there are concerns about the approach used to obtain the measurements. Thus, although the overall concept is interesting, there remains much to be done before this approach can be applied clinically. One looks forward to a more rigorous approach to determining physiological risk factors from data obtained by polysomnograms that might be useful clinically.

SYMPTOM SUBTYPES

Subjects with OSA also vary in the symptoms they complain of. There are distinct subtypes as revealed by unsupervised cluster analysis of data obtained from responses to a comprehensive questionnaire.[13] This was originally identified in the Icelandic Sleep Apnea Cohort.[13] The identified subtypes are the following: (1) disturbed sleep, that is, with symptoms of insomnia, (2) minimally symptomatic with minimal complaints related to their sleep or daytime function, and (3) excessive sleepiness. The latter subtype was less than 50% of the clinical cohort, and they were very sleepy with an average Epworth Sleepiness Score of more than 15.[13] Not surprisingly, subjects in the different symptom subtypes have different symptomatic benefits from continuous positive airway pressure (CPAP), with the excessively sleepy group obtaining the largest benefit.[14]

Although these clinical subtypes were originally identified in Iceland,[13] they have now been replicated in multiple clinical[15–17] and population-based[18–20] cohorts worldwide. When unsupervised clustering is applied in different cohorts, the optimal number of subtypes varies between 3 (as in Iceland) and 5. But the same 3 that were originally described are always present. In the Sleep Heart Health Study (SHHS), for example, the optimal solution is 4, that is, the original 3 plus a group with moderate sleepiness.[20] The prevalence of the different subtypes varies between clinical and population-based cohorts. For the latter, there

is, in general, a higher prevalence of the minimally symptomatic group. This is compatible with the assertion that OSA identified in population studies is different to that in subjects who present clinically.[21]

Although the existence of these subtypes is now well accepted, there are important unanswered questions. We currently do not know if individuals change subtype over time or remain in the same subtype. This is an important question that needs to be addressed before identification of symptomatic subtypes is used clinically.

Another important question is whether these subtypes have relevance to other outcomes of the disorder. Analysis in subjects in the SHHS found that an increased risk of cardiovascular outcomes only occurred in the excessively sleepy subtype but not the others.[20] This finding was replicated in a study in a clinical cohort in Chile.[15] This is compatible with an earlier observation that in elderly subjects with untreated OSA increased cardiovascular mortality only occurs in those with excessive sleepiness.[22] Similarly, in subjects who had a myocardial infarction and were found to have OSA, there was an increased rate of reinfarction in those who were excessively sleepy compared with those who were not.[23]

There are, however, studies that challenge the notion that there is an increased risk of CV events in those who are excessively sleepy.[16,24] It is not the sleepiness itself that confers risk. In the SHHS, there is no increased risk of CV events for those with sleepiness who do not have OSA.[20] The first negative study is from an investigation of 5358 patients with OSA in the Pays de la Laize cohort in France.[16] They identified the same 4 subgroups as in the SHHS but did not find that symptomatic subtypes at baseline were associated with future occurrence of major adverse CV events (MACE).[16] There is an association with OSA-specific hypoxic burden (HB) in the same subjects.[16]

In a subsequent study based on the same cohort, the benefit of CPAP treatment on CV outcomes was assessed.[25] They compared the rate of MACE on patients who did not use CPAP to those who did. Treating nonadherent patients as the reference group, they found that the adjusted hazard ratio (95% confidence intervals) for MACEs were 0.87 (0.73–1.04) for those using CPAP 4 to 6 hours on average per night, 0.75 (0.62–0.92) for those using CPAP more than 7 h/night. The findings were confirmed with a propensity score matching approach. The association was stronger in those who were excessively sleepy but the difference was not significant ($P = .060$).

Another study has recently been published that challenges the notion that those with excessive sleepiness are at increased risk for CV events.[24] This is based on a secondary analysis of the randomized Intervention with CPAP in CAD and OSA (RICCASDA) study, which assessed the benefit of CPAP on CV events in subjects with OSA who had coronary artery disease and were not excessively sleepy using a randomized design—CPAP or no CPAP.[26] In this analysis, they incorporated the excessively sleepy individuals who were not randomized. In the latter group, they compared outcomes in adherent to nonadherent subjects. They compared these results to data from the nonsleepy subjects in the RICCASDA trial. They found no differences in the defined CV outcomes by levels of sleepiness in subjects who were nonadherent to CPAP or untreated.[24] The sample sizes are small—155 who were excessively sleepy and 244 in the parent randomized trial. Thus, it is unclear how robust this negative result is.

One major difference between the several studies that showed that excessive sleepiness is associated with increased risk of CV events in subjects with OSA (see above) and those that did not is the use of CPAP. In studies showing this result, CPAP use was only in a small percentage of subjects while in the studies showing no effect, CPAP use was much higher. The use of CPAP in these studies makes interpretation more difficult. Nevertheless, it seems reasonable to assert that while this association is supported by several studies the jury is still out and other larger studies designed specifically to address this question are needed.

This is an important question to address. We have argued, based on the preponderance of the evidence, that the main reason that recent randomized controlled trials (RCTs) assessing the impact of CPAP on CV outcomes were negative is that they excluded subjects who were excessively sleepy.[27] In the largest study to date (the sleep apnea cardiovascular endpoints [SAVE] study[28]), the average Epworth Sleepiness Score of participants was 7.3 and 7.5 in the active and usual care group, respectively. The lack of inclusion of subjects with excessive sleepiness likely also affected the compliance to CPAP, which is lower in these RCTs than is described in patients being treated clinically.[29] Whether those with excessive sleepiness are at increased risk for CV events or not, there is no doubt that individuals recruited in these RCTs are not representative of the patients with OSA that are seen in sleep centers.[30] This issue is not specific to OSA and one of the challenges to RCTs is that they often study the "wrong people."[31]

NEW METRICS OF PHYSIOLOGICAL IMPACT OF OBSTRUCTIVE SLEEP APNEA

This question as to who with OSA is at an increased risk for adverse CV outcomes has prompted the development of new metrics of the disorder to assess whether they might be more predictive at future CV events than the apnea-hypopnea index.[32] Two new metrics have been developed. The first is HB.[33] It involves calculating the total desaturation area (**Fig. 1**) for each event and then summing all of these individual areas across the total period of sleep recording.[33] HB has been shown to be associated with cardiovascular mortality in the SHHS and the osteoporotic fractures in men (MrOS) population-based cohorts.[33] When analyses are repeated, however, in those with moderate-to-severe OSA in SHHS, no such association is found.[34] In the SHHS, HB is not associated with the occurrence of future nonfatal cardiovascular events but is with cardiovascular mortality.[34] Thus, it is conceivable that more intense hypoxia leads to fatal events during sleep. The time of occurrence of death in the SHHS is not currently available. In the SHHS and MrOS, HB also predicted future development of heart failure, whereas the apnea-hypopnea index did not.[35]

In the French clinical cohort, discussed above, HB was associated with the occurrence of cardiovascular events.[16] However, a retrospective analysis of data from the RICCASDA study in nonsleepy individuals did not find that HB predicted cardiovascular events or mortality.[36] Thus, the evidence that HB can be used to predict who is at increased risk for cardiovascular events is mixed. One challenge to using HB is that software to analyze data to obtain HB is, unfortunately, not open source. Philip de Chazel, at the University of Sydney, has developed an open source program to evaluate HB that will address this limitation.[34]

Although HB is not predictive of events in the RICCASDA study,[36] heart rate response to events is.[37] This measure assesses the degree of sudden increases in heart rate at the termination of events (**Fig. 2**). This is presumably a measure of the sympathetic response to events. There are 2 different implementations of this measure. In the first, it is related to arousals.[6] Heart rate response to arousals vary depending on the intensity of the arousal.[6] This varies among subjects; for example, heart rate response to arousal at a fixed intensity (eg, intensity 5) but within the same subject it is stable from night to night.[38] Twin studies show that the increase in heart rate response to arousals is heritable,[39] although the specific gene variants that are responsible are currently unknown. The alternative implementation is to ignore the issue

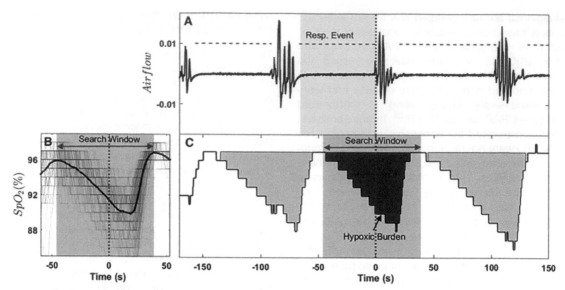

Fig. 1. The concept for calculation of hypoxic burden. The "area" of desaturation is calculated in a search window for each event. (Panel *A*) represents the flow signal with recurrent apneas; (Panel *B*) represents the method of calculation; (Panel *C*) is the desaturation area for repetitive events. (Reproduced with permission from ref.[33])

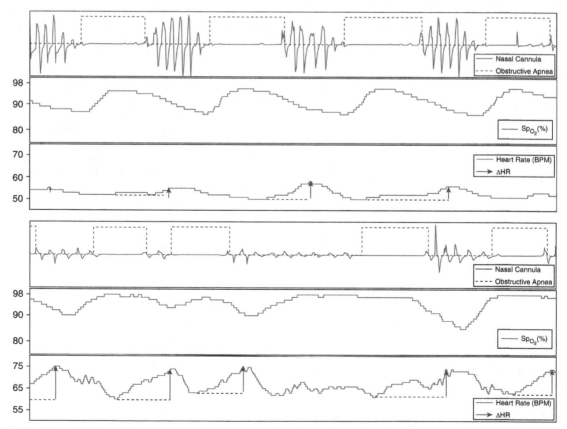

Fig. 2. The calculation of heart rate response to events. Two examples are shown with different magnitudes of heart rate response. (Reproduced with permission of the American Thoracic Society. Copyright © 2023 American Thoracic Society. All rights reserved. Azarbarzin A, Sands SA, Younes M, et al. The Sleep Apnea-Specific Pulse-Rate Response Predicts Cardiovascular Morbidity and Mortality. *Am J Respir Crit Care Med*. Jun 15 2021;203(12):1546-1555). The American Journal of Respiratory and Critical Care Medicine is an official journal of the American Thoracic Society.)

of intensity of arousal and simply evaluate the heart rate response to events, whether they be hypopneas or apneas. This has been applied to data collected in the Multi-Ethnic Study of Atherosclerosis (MESA) and in the SHHS.[40] In MESA, there is a U-shaped relationship between subclinical biomarkers of cardiovascular disease (CVD), for example, coronary calcification and heart rate response to events (ΔHR). In SHHS, individuals with high ΔHR were at increased risk of fatal and nonfatal CV events. The risk associated with a high ΔHR is particularly high in those with also a substantial HB and exclusively in those who are nonsleepy. In a retrospective analysis of the RIC-CASDA trial[26] in nonsleepy individuals with OSA and coronary artery disease, the CPAP-related reduction in risk of CV events/mortality increased progressively with the increasing ΔHR that was assessed before treatment was initiated.[37]

Thus, there is evidence that both HB and ΔHR are somewhat predictive of who is at increased risk of CV events. However, much more data are needed to fully assess the clinical value of these new measures.

SUMMARY

Throughout this brief review, we have emphasized that OSA is a heterogeneous disorder from multiple viewpoints. This represents a challenge and an opportunity. We need to assess the basis of these differences and their impact on diagnosis and management of patients. It seems unlikely that we will move away from CPAP being the first line of therapy. One immediate consequence of these studies is to question whether all subjects with OSA need to be treated. It has been argued that all of those who are minimally symptomatic may not require treatment.[41] An algorithm has been proposed, which requires additional testing to assess if a subgroup of such subjects might benefit from therapy.[41] Others have proposed, however, that this should not be our focus given the relative lack of clinical resources for diagnosis and treatment of OSA.[42] Rather, we should focus on identifying those who are excessively sleepy.[42] They are known to benefit symptomatically from CPAP treatment,[14] and it is likely, although not certain, that they will also have a benefit in terms of reduction of future CV events (see above). Although currently there are studies documenting the rate of undiagnosed OSA,[43,44] we do not know what subtype such subjects belong to. This is an important question to address. If these undiagnosed subjects are largely in the minimally symptomatic group, the rate of undiagnosed OSA is not as concerning.

CLINICS CARE POINTS

- Endotypes of sleep apnea have been identified but determining them in clinical use is challenging.
- There are different symptomatic subtypes of OSA.
- There is a question as to whether minimally symptomatic patients with OSA require treatment.

There are new metrics of the physiological derangements that are secondary to OSA, that is, HB and heart rate response to events. They have an association with future cardiovascular events/mortality.

DISCLOSURE

The author has nothing to disclose.

ACKNOWLEDGMENTS

Funding was provided by NIH, United States grant P01 HL094307.

REFERENCES

1. Benjafield AV, Ayas NT, Eastwood PR, et al. Estimation of the global prevalence and burden of obstructive sleep apnoea: a literature-based analysis. Lancet Respir Med 2019;7(8):687–98.
2. Wellman A, Eckert DJ, Jordan AS, et al. A method for measuring and modeling the physiological traits causing obstructive sleep apnea. J Appl Physiol 2011;110(6):1627–37.
3. Edwards BA, Sands SA, Owens RL, et al. The combination of supplemental oxygen and a hypnotic markedly improves obstructive sleep apnea in patients with a mild to moderate upper airway collapsibility. Sleep 2016;39(11):1973–83.
4. Terrill PI, Edwards BA, Nemati S, et al. Quantifying the ventilatory control contribution to sleep apnoea using polysomnography. Eur Respir J 2015;45(2):408–18.
5. Younes M, Schwab R. Con: Can physiological risk factors for obstructive sleep apnea be determined by analysis of data obtained from routine polysomnography? Sleep 2023;46(5):zsac158.
6. Azarbarzin A, Ostrowski M, Hanly P, et al. Relationship between arousal intensity and heart rate response to arousal. Sleep 2014;37(4):645–53.
7. Sands SA, Edwards BA. Pro: Can physiological risk factors for obstructive sleep apnea be determined

by analysis of data obtained from routine polysom-nography? Sleep 2023;46(5):zsac310.

8. Alex RM, Sofer T, Azarbarzin A, et al. Within-night repeatability and long-term consistency of sleep apnea endotypes: the multi-ethnic study of atherosclerosis and osteoporotic fractures in men study. Sleep 2022;45(9):zsac129.

9. Magalang UJ, Grant BJB. Understanding stability of obstructive sleep apnea endotypes: a step forward. Sleep 2022;45(9):zsac174.

10. Won CHJ, Reid M, Sofer T, et al. Sex differences in obstructive sleep apnea phenotypes, the multi-ethnic study of atherosclerosis. Sleep 2020;43(5):zsz274.

11. Bamagoos AA, Cistulli PA, Sutherland K, et al. Polysomnographic endotyping to select patients with obstructive sleep apnea for oral appliances. Ann Am Thorac Soc 2019;16(11):1422–31.

12. Op de Beeck S, Dieltjens M, Azarbarzin A, et al. Mandibular advancement device treatment efficacy is associated with polysomnographic endotypes. Ann Am Thorac Soc 2021;18(3):511–8.

13. Ye L, Pien GW, Ratcliffe SJ, et al. The different clinical faces of obstructive sleep apnoea: a cluster analysis. Eur Respir J 2014;44(6):1600–7.

14. Pien GW, Ye L, Keenan BT, et al. Changing faces of obstructive sleep apnea: treatment effects by cluster designation in the Icelandic Sleep Apnea Cohort. Sleep 2018;41(3):zsx201.

15. Labarca G, Dreyse J, Salas C, et al. A clinic-based cluster analysis in patients with moderate-severe obstructive sleep apnea (OSA) in Chile. Sleep Med 2020;73:16–22.

16. Trzepizur W, Blanchard M, Ganem T, et al. Sleep apnea-specific hypoxic burden, symptom subtypes, and risk of cardiovascular events and all-cause mortality. Am J Respir Crit Care Med 2022;205(1):108–17.

17. Keenan BT, Kim J, Singh B, et al. Recognizable clinical subtypes of obstructive sleep apnea across international sleep centers: a cluster analysis. Sleep 2018;41(3):zsx214.

18. Kim J, Keenan BT, Lim DC, et al. Symptom-based subgroups of Koreans with obstructive sleep apnea. J Clin Sleep Med 2018;14(3):437–43.

19. Gonzalez KA, Tarraf W, Wallace DM, et al. Phenotypes of obstructive sleep apnea in the hispanic community Health study/study of latinos. Sleep 2021;44(12):zsab181.

20. Mazzotti DR, Keenan BT, Lim DC, et al. Symptom subtypes of obstructive sleep apnea predict incidence of cardiovascular outcomes. Am J Respir Crit Care Med 2019;200(4):493–506.

21. Arnardottir ES, Bjornsdottir E, Olafsdottir KA, et al. Obstructive sleep apnoea in the general population: highly prevalent but minimal symptoms. Eur Respir J 2016;47(1):194–202.

22. Gooneratne NS, Richards KC, Joffe M, et al. Sleep disordered breathing with excessive daytime sleepiness is a risk factor for mortality in older adults. Sleep 2011;34(4):435–42.

23. Xie J, Sert Kuniyoshi FH, Covassin N, et al. Excessive daytime sleepiness independently predicts increased cardiovascular risk after myocardial infarction. J Am Heart Assoc 2018;7(2):e007221.

24. Eulenburg C, Celik Y, Redline S, et al. Cardiovascular outcomes in adults with coronary artery disease and obstructive sleep apnea with vs without excessive daytime sleepiness in the RICCADSA cohort. Ann Am Thorac Soc 2023. https://doi.org/10.1513/AnnalsATS.202208-676OC.

25. Gerves-Pinquie C, Bailly S, Goupil F, et al. Positive airway pressure adherence, mortality and cardiovascular events in sleep apnea patients. Am J Respir Crit Care Med 2022;206(11). 1393-1140.

26. Peker Y, Glantz H, Eulenburg C, et al. Effect of positive airway pressure on cardiovascular outcomes in coronary artery disease patients with nonsleepy obstructive sleep apnea. The RICCADSA randomized controlled trial. Am J Respir Crit Care Med 2016;194(5):613–20.

27. Pack AI, Magalang UJ, Singh B, et al. Randomized clinical trials of cardiovascular disease in obstructive sleep apnea: understanding and overcoming bias. Sleep 2021;44(2):zsaa229.

28. McEvoy RD, Antic NA, Heeley E, et al. CPAP for prevention of cardiovascular events in obstructive sleep apnea. Multicenter Study Randomized Controlled Trial. N Engl J Med 2016;375(10):919–31.

29. Cistulli PA, Armitstead J, Pepin JL, et al. Short-term CPAP adherence in obstructive sleep apnea: a big data analysis using real world data. Sleep Med 2019;59:114–6.

30. Reynor A, McArdle N, Shenoy B, et al. Continuous positive airway pressure and adverse cardiovascular events in obstructive sleep apnea: are participants of randomized trials representative of sleep clinic patients? Sleep 2022;45(4):zsab264.

31. Lauer MS, Gordon D, Wei G, et al. Efficient design of clinical trials and epidemiological research: is it possible? Nat Rev Cardiol 2017;14(8):493–501.

32. Malhotra A, Ayappa I, Ayas N, et al. Metrics of sleep apnea severity: beyond the apnea-hypopnea index. Sleep 2021;44(7):zsab030.

33. Azarbarzin A, Sands SA, Stone KL, et al. The hypoxic burden of sleep apnoea predicts cardiovascular disease-related mortality: the Osteoporotic Fractures in Men Study and the Sleep Heart Health Study. Eur Heart J 2019;40(14):1149–57.

34. Mazzotti DR, Magalang UJ, Keenan BT, et al. OSA symptom subtypes and hypoxic burden independently predict distinct cardiovascular outcomes. Sleep 2023 (in revision).

35. Azarbarzin A, Sands SA, Taranto-Montemurro L, et al. The sleep apnea-specific hypoxic burden

predicts incident heart failure. Chest 2020;158(2): 739–50.

36. Azarbarzin A, Zinchuk A, Peker Y, et al. Reply to: heart rate response in obstructive sleep apnea: a clue to reveal cardiovascular benefit from continuous positive airway pressure? Am J Respir Crit Care Med 2022;206(9):1181–2.

37. Azarbarzin A, Zinchuk A, Wellman A, et al. Cardiovascular benefit of continuous positive airway pressure in adults with coronary artery disease and obstructive sleep apnea without excessive sleepiness. Am J Respir Crit Care Med 2022;206(6): 767–74.

38. Azarbarzin A, Ostrowski M, Younes M, et al. Arousal responses during overnight polysomnography and their reproducibility in healthy young adults. Sleep 2015;38(8):1313–21.

39. Gao X, Azarbarzin A, Keenan BT, et al. Heritability of heart rate response to arousals in twins. Sleep 2017; 40(6). https://doi.org/10.1093/sleep/zsx055.

40. Azarbarzin A, Sands SA, Younes M, et al. The sleep apnea-specific pulse-rate response predicts cardiovascular morbidity and mortality. Am J Respir Crit Care Med 2021;203(12):1546–55.

41. Pengo MF, Gozal D, Martinez-Garcia MA. Should we treat with continuous positive airway pressure severe non-sleepy obstructive sleep apnea individuals without underlying cardiovascular disease? Sleep 2022;45(12):zsac208.

42. Donovan LM, Patel SR. Approaching sleep apnea management in the setting of uncertainty. Sleep 2022;45(12):zsac234.

43. Arsic B, Zebic K, Sajid A, et al. Assessing the adequacy of obstructive sleep apnea diagnosis for high-risk patients in primary care. J Am Board Fam Med : JABFM 2022;35(2):320–8.

44. Heffner JE, Rozenfeld Y, Kai M, et al. Prevalence of diagnosed sleep apnea among patients with type 2 diabetes in primary care. Chest 2012;141(6): 1414–21.

Creating an Optimal Approach for Diagnosing Sleep Apnea

Jean-Louis Pépin, MD, PhD[a,b,*], Renaud Tamisier, MD, PhD[a,b],
Sébastien Baillieul, MD, PhD[a,b], Raoua Ben Messaoud, PhD[a,b],
Alison Foote, PhD[b], Sébastien Bailly, PharmD, PhD[a,b],
Jean-Benoît Martinot, MD[c,d]

KEYWORDS

- Sleep apnea • Diagnosis • Home sleep apnea testing • Virtual sleep laboratory
- Mandibular jaw movements • Photoplethysmography • Peripheral arterial tone

KEY POINTS

- Home multi-night sleep testing reduces misclassification of sleep apnea level of severity.
- Scoring of abnormal respiratory events and sleep disturbances could be assisted by artificial intelligence to reduce burden of manual scoring and inter-scorer variability.
- Sleep testing methods should be low-cost, simple to install, and easy to use at home.
- Robust clinical trials are needed to validate new sensors, algorithms, and digital solutions.

INTRODUCTION

Sleep apnea is one of the most frequent chronic diseases, affecting nearly one billion people worldwide.[1] Its prevalence is expected to continue to increase owing to the sustained progression of obesity, sedentariness, and diabetes epidemics that represent the most common risk factors for sleep apnea.[2] At an individual level, sleep apnea is responsible for deterioration in quality of life, neurocognitive dysfunctions, and sleepiness (causing related traffic accidents).[3,4] Sleep apnea is associated with a higher risk of the occurrence and cumulation of cardiometabolic comorbidities, which in turn lead to early mortality.[5–7] The impact on health systems is substantial, and in response to the burden of sleep apnea, specific national programs have been initiated to review diagnostic methods, along with the reorganization of treatment and follow-up care pathways.[8]

Conventionally, diagnosis usually depends on overnight polysomnography in a sleep clinic, for which there are often long waiting lists, as well as being highly human-resource intensive. Once diagnosed, the efficient treatments are available to confront the medical challenge of sleep apnea. Continuous positive airway pressure (CPAP) is the first-line therapy for moderate-to-severe obstructive sleep apnea (OSA) and is highly efficient in improving quality of life and reducing symptoms and sleepiness.[9] The efficacy of CPAP is less clear concerning reduction in the risk of cardiovascular diseases and mortality, but there is strong evidence from real-word studies of a positive impact[10,11] of OSA treatment. Positive airway therapies also reduce health-related costs, particularly in the comorbid combinations of sleep apnea and chronic obstructive pulmonary disease (COPD),[12] or sleep apnea and type 2 diabetes.[13]

Although often ignored in the past, for all these reasons there is an increase in sleep apnea

[a] Univ. Grenoble Alpes, HP2 (Hypoxia and Physio-Pathologies) Laboratory, Inserm (French National Institute of Health and Medical Research) U1300, Grenoble, 38000 France; [b] Sleep Laboratory, Grenoble Alpes University Hospital Center, Grenoble, 38043 France; [c] Sleep Laboratory, CHU Université Catholique de Louvain (UCL) Namur Site Sainte-Elisabeth, Namur, Belgium; [d] Institute of Experimental and Clinical Research, UCL Bruxelles Woluwe, Brussels, Belgium
* Corresponding author. Laboratoire EFCR, CHU de Grenoble Alpes, CS10217, 38043, Grenoble.
E-mail address: JPepin@chu-grenoble.fr

Sleep Med Clin 18 (2023) 301–309
https://doi.org/10.1016/j.jsmc.2023.05.004

awareness among health care professionals, health insurers, and individuals having risk factors of sleep apnea. Therefore, in recent years, there has been a huge increase in the demand for sleep apnea diagnosis and treatment pathway workflows. For example, a national registry study in Finland reported a continuous increase in the societal burden caused by sleep apnea over the last 20 years, constant progression in outpatient visits in primary and secondary care and an increase in the cumulative annual number of days off work for sleep apnea.[8] In the Finnish case, to meet these growing demands, diagnostic methods were simplified and more often conducted in an ambulatory setting, treatment pathways were revised, and patient follow-up was reorganized. Consequently, despite a remarkable increase in the number of patients, there was a significant decrease in societal costs per patient.[8] This is a pragmatic demonstration that the urgently needed reforms in sleep apnea diagnosis and treatment workflow are feasible, benefiting both patients and society as a whole.[14,15]

Advances to Be Made in Sleep Apnea Diagnosis

This review aims to summarize the main improvements that could be made in sleep apnea diagnosis. We do not discuss sleep apnea symptoms or specific clinical contexts. Several major issues are addressed.

1. Patients and caregivers share expectations for the rapid deployment of simplified and home sleep testing. Multi-night assessment certainly represents the future, avoiding misclassification of sleep apnea level of severity.
2. The introduction of novel technologies and sensors (after appropriate validation as medical devices) or end-to-end diagnostic solutions is necessary.
3. Scoring of abnormal respiratory events and sleep disturbances should be supported by automated devices and interpretable artificial intelligence.
4. New approaches to sleep apnea diagnosis should be appropriate to meet the size of the epidemiologic problem. Testing methods should be low-cost and easy-to-use to allow dissemination *at all scales* in diverse health systems.

Multi-Night Home Sleep Apnea Testing

The American Academy of Sleep Medicine has established clinical practice guidelines supporting home sleep apnea testing (HSAT) with technically adequate devices for the diagnosis of OSA in "uncomplicated adult patients presenting with signs and symptoms that indicate an increased risk of moderate to severe OSA" (Strong Recommendation).[16] In patients with a high pretest probability of OSA without unstable comorbidities, comorbid insomnia, or suspicion of nocturnal hypoventilation, HSAT now represents the standard of care in many countries.

However, it is currently widely accepted that for patients with mild-to-moderate sleep apnea, a single night of polysomnography or HSAT can lead to misclassification of disease severity in nearly one-third of patients. This is explained by the substantial night-to-night variability in the apnea–hypopnea index (AHI)[17–19] and unevenness in sleep quality.[20] Also, up to 21% of patients might be overdiagnosed, whereas 7% might be underdiagnosed based on a single-night AHI value.[21] In-laboratory sleep studies probably exacerbate misclassifications when compared with at-home measurements as place and type of recording are modulating factors susceptible to influencing the AHI. The "first night effect" is probably higher in the sleep laboratory owing to the unusual sleep environment leading in turn to changes in sleep architecture, different sleep positions, and consequently variations in respiratory event indices.[17] Sleep body position is largely determined by the recording device used, as some devices affect the ability to sleep in a lateral decubitus position.

In summary, among the current requirements for an accurate diagnostic workup of OSA, it is now time that at-home multi-night testing becomes mainstream practice.[22] Such a multi-night sleep testing strategy has been challenged due to potentially higher health care costs and greater inconvenience to patients. However, newly available digital medicine end-to-end diagnostic solutions will significantly simplify at-home multi-night testing allowing efficient cost-effective diagnostic pathways to be implemented.[21,23–27]

Knowledge Gaps and Research Perspectives

Number of nights of sleep testing

The number of nights of sleep testing required for a reliable and accurate OSA diagnosis is still under debate.[22,28,29] The optimum number of nights required is a compromise between the inconvenience for the patient, cost-effectiveness, and the precision required for clinical decision-making. Most of the studies addressing night-to-night variability in AHI have been conducted over two or three consecutive nights. Recently, Lechat and colleagues[21] have amassed an impressive amount of home sleep data to describe the variability and misclassification of OSA. Using a noninvasive under-mattress sensor technology, 67,278 individuals aged between 18 and 90 years underwent in-home nightly monitoring over an average of approximately 170 nights per participant.[21] The main "inflection" point of the number of nights versus diagnostic confidence curves occurs between 5 and 10 nights, after which there is only a relatively small improvement in diagnostic performance.[29] Undertreatment probability drops to 14% and overtreatment to 6% with a 5-night diagnostic test corresponding to an approximately twofold increase in overall diagnostic performance.[29]

The number of nights required is probably also related to the diagnostic performance of the diagnosis tool used and the typology of patients. Some sleep apnea phenotypes are associated with higher AHI variability, particularly mild-to-moderate OSA, OSA with comorbid insomnia and/or cardiovascular diseases, and behavioral and lifestyle factors such as alcohol consumption. A pragmatic view might be to start with 5 nights for all patients and in case of large night-to-night variability, extend to 7 to 10 nights.

Apnea–hypopnea index variability: A new metric for sleep apnea diagnosis and clinical decision-making

Sole reliance on the AHI for the classification of OSA severity has been challenged[30] as it may not precisely reflect the OSA-related hypoxic burden and acute cardiovascular responses that are the best predictors of long-term hard outcomes and mortality.[11] In the quest for metrics to better characterize OSA severity and to guide therapeutic decisions, information gained by multi-night recordings might change practices. It is unknown whether the mean, median, or standard deviation of AHI will be a better predictor of outcomes. This question has been recently nicely addressed for atrial fibrillation[31] and the occurrence of malignant ventricular arrhythmias in heart failure patients appropriately treated with implantable cardioverter-defibrillators.[32] There was a significant association between the variability in sleep-disordered breathing recorded over several nights and the number of appropriate shocks. Very recently, it has been shown that a single-night assessment of OSA failed to detect any association with hypertension. Conversely, the association with hypertension was clearly detected when AHI was measured over ≥28 nights.[33] These details are of fundamental importance when aiming to develop risk prediction analyses or performing clinical trials in the OSA field. Also, studies assessing the link between the variability of AHI

at diagnosis and simple clinical outcomes such as excessive daytime sleepiness, quality of life, or long-term CPAP adherence are missing so far.

Implementation of Novel Technologies, Sensors, and End-to-End Solutions

Polysomnography provides three main categories of information required for accurate sleep apnea diagnosis (Fig. 1): sleep characterization (ie, architecture, microstructure, and fragmentation); number and nature of respiratory events (ie, apneas, hypopneas, respiratory effort-related arousals, and central vs obstructive components); and acute cardiorespiratory responses (ie, sympathetic activity and hypoxic burden). To capture all these data, multiple sensors are needed requiring long installation times, specialized technical expertise for scoring, and continuous monitoring during the night of the multiple recording channels by a sleep professional. Automated scoring of polysomnography has been introduced to ease the task of sleep technicians and render the scoring more objective.[34,35]

A major step forward for the easy implementation and smooth running of new diagnostic procedures would be to validate and render available a limited number of innovative sensors and metrics, able to summarize all the information needed to determine sleep disorder pathophysiology and classify disease severity. Indeed, a plethora of technologies has emerged to diagnose sleep apnea in the home setting. Mandibular jaw movements (MJMs),[23–25,36] photoplethysmography (PPG), and peripheral arterial tone[26,37] are among the most promising techniques that have already been shown to perform well in different research and clinical settings.

Mandibular Jaw Movements

There are new technologies for detecting and recording MJM in the home setting. A sensor taped on the chin captures inertial energy in a three-dimensional system of measurement providing data from a total of six derived channels (Sunrise).[23–25] At a given point in time, some channels are more informative than others depending on the position of the body, head, and mandible.

The mandibular jaw plays the role of a prop stabilizing the pharynx, ensuring upper airway patency, and reducing upper airway resistance in the presence of negative and suctioning pressure inside the airways during inspiration. MJMs reflect both respiratory drive and variations in the respiratory effort (RE), which typically occur during abnormal respiratory events. This reliable measurement of respiratory drive/effort allows an

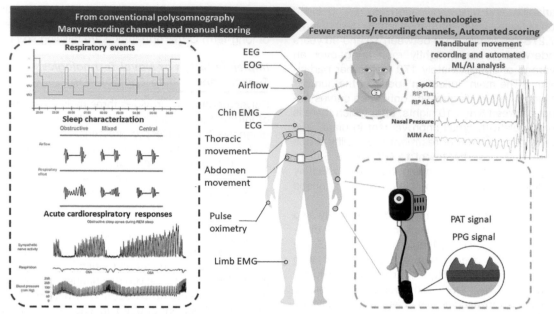

Fig. 1. Transition from the conventional sleep apnea diagnostic pathway based on overnight polysomnography in a sleep clinic to home multi-night testing based on new innovative sensors and digital solutions. Polysomnography (PSG) in a sleep clinic includes many different recording channels: brain activity (EEG), eye movements (EOG), muscle activity (EMG), heart rhythm (ECG), abdominal movement (ABD), and so forth. Home sleep testing has fewer recording channels: mandibular jaw movements (MJM), peripheral arterial tonometry (PAT), and photoplethysmography (PPG).

accurate identification of obstructive versus central events[38] and a unique characterization of the cumulative burden of RE throughout the night.[36]

MJMs are the net result of the activation of brainstem respiratory and sleep centers and their respective interactions.[24] This interaction modulates the amplitude and frequency of MJM across the different sleep stages allowing sleep staging.[24] During light sleep (N2), the amplitude of MJM is of several tenths of a millimeter and varies slightly. The amplitude of MJM increases during normal deepening of sleep into non-rapid eye movement sleep (N3) when upper airway resistance is known to increase. N3 MJM is also more stable than during N2. Rapid eye movement (REM) sleep is easily identified by irregular frequencies and changing amplitudes in MJM reflecting tonic and phasic sleep. MJM amplitudes during REM are on average smaller than non-REM sleep amplitudes.

At present, the only known limitation of MJM is difficulty in fixing the sensor to the chin of men with abundant beards.

Photoplethysmography and peripheral arterial tonometry

PPG and peripheral arterial tonometry (PAT) are noninvasive measurements reflecting sympathetic activity. PPG measures small variations in light absorption associated with changes in tissue perfusion, usually at the fingertip.[39] The pulsatile component of the waveform reflects changes in blood volume occurring with each heartbeat and the amplitude between pulsatile changes reflects autonomic tone.[39] PAT measures the pulsatile arterial volume at the finger, which depends on sympathetic activity, providing a window into the autonomic nervous system.

Most respiratory events in sleep apnea end in cortical and/or autonomic arousals leading to peripheral sympathetic activation. Intrinsically, PAT and PPG signals have the potential to identify micro-arousals associated with these surges in sympathetic activity ending the respiratory events. Sympathetic activation causes vasoconstriction and heart rate acceleration resulting in attenuation of the PAT and PPG signals. The interval between micro-arousals then corresponds to the frequency of respiratory events. The combination with other signals, such as SaO_2, snoring, and thoracic impedance, can improve performances and complete PAT and PPG information. In addition, measurement of the tonic and phasic sympathetic tones and their variations also allows an estimation of sleep stages and total sleep time.

The combination of simultaneous assessment of PAT/PPG with two or three additional signals (including SaO_2) allows us to derive a comprehensive characterization of sleep architecture and the main indices of sleep apnea severity. Two devices integrated into digital solutions are already available on the market (ie, WatchPAT and NightOwl). They work with acceptable levels of performances.[37,40] However, misclassification can occur for mild- and moderate-severity classes of sleep apnea, whereas the recognition of severe sleep apnea is good. Once again (see paragraph above), use over multiple nights represents a solution to increase the robustness of these ambulatory home-based diagnostic tools.

Automated Devices and Artificial Intelligence for Scoring Respiratory Events and Sleep Disturbances

The manual scoring of respiratory and sleep events requires expert specialist staff and is very time- and human-resource-consuming. Moreover, manual scoring and the classification of sleep epochs have two essential drawbacks.

Manual scoring is associated with large intra- and inter-scorer variability

This significant limitation persists even in well-trained teams and despite well-established scoring criteria. In a recent study,[25] we compared home sleep testing using mandibular movements (MJMs) with at-home polysomnography that was blindly scored by two expert centers (in Grenoble and London). There was significant variability among the experienced experts (ie, inter-scorer agreement reached only 80%) despite the use of standardized scoring criteria. These discrepancies have been known for many years and are present even in centers with highly trained staff.[41] The magnitude of this difference between centers was similar to the difference between the machine learning automated scoring of MJMs compared with the respiratory disturbance index calculated from both the Grenoble and London PSG manual scorings. This demonstrates that the automatic scoring of sleep and respiratory events offers many advantages beyond simply a reduction in the human resources needed for routine manual scoring and a reduction in the subjectivity associated with manual scoring. Overall, automated algorithms for scoring sleep and respiratory events have now achieved an acceptable level of accuracy and agreement close to 85% with manual scoring.[42] A common strategy being introduced in the routine practice of many sleep laboratories is to start with automated scoring followed by an auto-edited approach, especially when there are inconsistencies between pretest probability and the results of the automated scoring.

Epoch-Based Manual Scoring Fails to Capture Much Information Contained in the Signals

The recognition of a respiratory event limited to preestablished criteria leads to an artificial disconnection between interlinked physiologic and pathophysiologic events with the loss of the understanding of temporal links or the dynamics of specific event trajectories. This reduces the richness of the physiologic signals available with the loss of important information relevant to the patient's diagnostic characterization and therapeutic decision-making. It is now well known that AHI is not the perfect metric for sleep-disordered breathing[29] and is poorly correlated with outcomes. Other, previously often overlooked quantifiable overall features within polysomnographic data such as the hypoxic burden or acute cardiovascular responses to respiratory events have recently been demonstrated as being more strongly related to poor prognosis than AHI.[30] No doubt, in the near future, diagnostic nights will include metrics more representative of what is truly related to symptoms, quality of life, and hard outcomes. Current conventional scoring does not capture the cumulative burden of sympathetic tone, sleep microstructure, and RE, all key consequences of the repetitive occurrence of respiratory events during sleep. Overnight sympathetic tone is possible to capture by PPG and PAT signals and we need studies showing the impact of the cumulative elevation in sympathetic activity during the night on hard outcomes in the context of OSA. It has been recently demonstrated that fine-tuning microstructure changes (ie, slow-wave activity and sleep spindles) allow the identification of indices that are strong predictors of incident hypertension.[43] Increased RE is one of the main features of OSA and is associated with sympathetic overactivity, leading to increased vascular wall stiffness and remodeling. We have recently demonstrated that the proportion of sleep time spent with increased RE (automatically derived from MJM by machine learning analyses) is potentially a reliable new metric to predict prevalent hypertension in patients with OSA.[36]

Automation and interpretable artificial intelligence

Overall, it appears obvious that algorithmic metrics and artificial intelligence have the capabilities to enrich diagnosis and support risk prediction in OSA by conveying more information than classical PSG metrics. They will provide metrics that reflect more accurately the sleep-related dynamics of disease burden and the associated risks. To convince the sleep community, and in particular

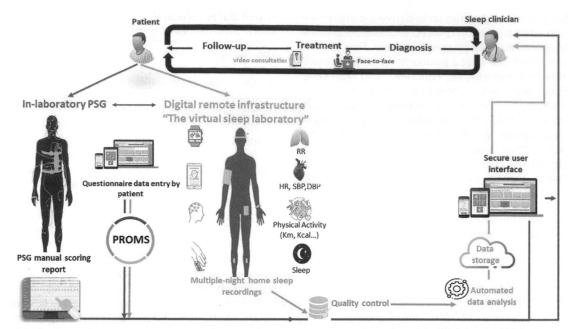

Fig. 2. The place of digital solutions in the sleep apnea diagnostic pathway. The virtual sleep laboratory would collect measurements made by the patient themselves or with the help of a carer, nurse, or sleep technician, such as patient reported outcome measures (PROMS), respiratory rate (RR), heart rate (HR), blood pressure (SBP and DBP), physical activity, daytime sleepiness, self-reported sleep disturbance, and then data from home sleep tests over several nights using innovative sensors. Comorbidities might necessitate a conventional polysomnography. Data could initially be analyzed using automated ML algorithms with recourse to the sleep clinician when in doubt. The treatment decision should be made at a face-to-face or video consultation with the sleep physician in the light of all available data. DPB, diastolic blood pressure; ML, machine learning; SBP, systolic blood pressure.

clinicians, of their relevance and value algorithmic codes and software should be made readily available, open access, and easily sharable between laboratories worldwide to allow replicability. Machine learning and artificial intelligence are powerful tools but are often considered "black box" methods due to their complexity, generating disillusionment and distrust. It is crucial that the models and outputs remain reasonably interpretable by sleep experts in terms of physiologic and pathophysiologic patterns.[44] Direct collaborations between the end users (clinicians), and the target audience (patients) in model conception and development are mandatory and will increase trustworthiness and hence dissemination in the field. It is a new challenge for scientific sleep societies to propose a set of best practices for validation studies and guidelines regarding the use of these tools and the new metrics they generate. Accordingly, a recent systematic review found that despite the large number of medical machine learning-based algorithms and digital tools in development for medicine, only a few randomized controlled trials (RCTs) of rather low quality have been conducted for these technologies.[45]

New Diagnostic Approaches Appropriate to the Size of the Epidemiologic Problem

Despite the potential of innovative diagnostic pathways to improve multiple aspects of patient care, barriers to their large-scale clinical adoption exist. There is a need to reinvent not only the diagnosis tools but also the patient's complete journey from suspicion of OSA to long-term treatment follow-up. For the workup of patients suspected of sleep apnea, technological innovation should certainly be introduced in the form of a remote digital infrastructure, often called a "virtual sleep laboratory"[27] (**Fig. 2**). The virtual sleep laboratory would propose preliminary screening with, if appropriate, a recommendation for a home sleep test (ideally over multiple nights), data collection, and interpretation in a digital pipeline, strictly following data privacy rules. This type of framework should also propose an initial clinical evaluation that includes appropriate patient-reported outcomes as these will contribute to compliance with therapy. A second virtual or face-to-face consultation would allow treatment decision-making shared with the patient and inclusion in the treatment follow-up management pathway. A specialized nurse or sleep technician could supervise quality control and the progress of the patients through the diagnostic pathway and ensure that the sleep physician has access to home sleep test results for the final treatment decision. Complex cases, including patients with comorbidities, might be directly redirected to the classical diagnostic pathway of in-laboratory evaluation after the first consultation or after home sleep testing. Although such an organization is highly attractive to improve access to sleep apnea diagnosis, there are two major issues to address. First, the governance and management of these virtual infrastructures should certainly remain under the supervision of board-certified sleep physicians rather than private companies. Second, the dissemination of these digital solutions will push national health agencies to find new reimbursement models covering all aspects of the diagnostic pathways and not each activity separately (ie, consultations, HSAT) throughout the diagnostic workflow. Some studies have already examined the feasibility of such approaches and patient satisfaction. For example, virtual management has been evaluated in atrial fibrillation outpatient clinics[27] showing a shorter time to diagnosis and high patient satisfaction. Of note, previously undiagnosed sleep apnea was frequently detected and the patient prescribed sleep-disordered breathing treatments in association with atrial fibrillation ablation.[27]

CONCLUSION AND PERSPECTIVES

The increase in awareness and knowledge about sleep apnea among both the general public and health professionals necessitates a quick and effective response to meet the growth in demand for health care services dedicated to the diagnosis and follow-up of OSA patients.[15,46] In this review, we have identified new initiatives, key areas for further research, gaps in our knowledge, and issues to be solved before being able to translate and scale up promising innovations into routine practice. The expansion and dissemination of these new technologies into clinical settings require greater communication between sleep medicine experts, sleep-learned societies, and companies. It is the role of policymakers and the scientific community to ask for a robust demonstration of performance and cost-effectiveness in improving key patient-centered outcomes.[34,47] There is a potential that the implementation of digital technology and cloud-based analysis and data sharing will foster complementarity and interchange between conventional sleep laboratories and virtual sleep laboratories, improving access to care and reducing health care fragmentation.

CLINICS CARE POINTS

- New technologies should permit diagnostic sleep tests to be performed over several nights at home.
- Night-to-night variability in the apnea–hypopnea index should be included in obstructive sleep apnea severity classification.
- Alongside and in addition to classical sleep laboratories the "virtual sleep laboratory" should be developed.

DISCLOSURE

J.L. Pepin and J.B. Martinot are non-remunerated scientific advisors to Sunrise. J.L. Pepin has received research grants and consultancy fees from Itamar Medical. None of the other authors have a conflict of interest with respect to this review.

FUNDING

French National Research Agency (ANR) in the framework of the "Investissements d'avenir" program (ANR-15-IDEX-02) and the Grenoble Alpes University Foundation chairs of excellence: "e-health and integrated care and trajectories medicine" and "MIAI artificial intelligence." This work has been partially supported by the Grenoble Alpes Multidisciplinary Institute in Artificial Intelligence (MIAI) (ANR-19-P3IA-0003).

REFERENCES

1. Benjafield AV, Ayas NT, Eastwood PR, et al. Estimation of the global prevalence and burden of obstructive sleep apnoea: a literature-based analysis. Lancet Respir Med 2019;7(8):687–98.
2. Hudgel DW, Patel SR, Ahasic AM, et al. The role of weight management in the treatment of adult obstructive sleep apnea. An official American thoracic society clinical practice guideline. Am J Respir Crit Care Med 2018;198(6):e70–87.
3. Rosenzweig I, Glasser M, Polsek D, et al. Sleep apnoea and the brain: a complex relationship. Lancet Respir Med 2015;3(5):404–14.
4. Lal C, Ayappa I, Ayas N, et al. The link between obstructive sleep apnea and neurocognitive impairment: an official American thoracic society workshop report. Ann Am Thorac Soc 2022;19(8): 1245–56.

5. Ryan S, Cummins EP, Farre R, et al. Understanding the pathophysiological mechanisms of cardiometabolic complications in obstructive sleep apnoea: towards personalized treatment approaches. Eur Respir J 2020;56(2):1902295.

6. Lévy P, Kohler M, McNicholas WT, et al. Obstructive sleep apnoea syndrome. Nat Rev Dis Primers 2015; 1:15015.

7. Yeghiazarians Y, Jneid H, Tietjens JR, et al. Obstructive sleep apnea and cardiovascular disease: a scientific statement from the American heart association. Circulation 2021;144(3).e56–67.

8. Mattila T, Hasala H, Kreivi HR, et al. Changes in the societal burden caused by sleep apnoea in Finland from 1996 to 2018: a national registry study. Lancet Reg Health Eur 2022;16:100338.

9. Li Z, Cai S, Wang J, et al. Predictors of the efficacy for daytime sleepiness in patients with obstructive sleep apnea with continual positive airway pressure therapy: a meta-analysis of randomized controlled trials. Front Neurol 2022;13:911996.

10. Pépin JL, Bailly S, Rinder P, et al. Relationship between CPAP termination and all-cause mortality: a French nationwide database analysis. Chest 2022; 161(6):1657–65.

11. Gervès-Pinquié C, Bailly S, Goupil F, et al. Positive airway pressure adherence, mortality, and cardiovascular events in patients with sleep apnea. Am J Respir Crit Care Med 2022;206(11):1393–404.

12. Sterling KL, Pépin JL, Linde-Zwirble W, et al. Impact of positive airway pressure therapy adherence on outcomes in patients with obstructive sleep apnea and chronic obstructive pulmonary disease. Am J Respir Crit Care Med 2022;206(2):197–205.

13. Sterling KL, Cistulli PA, Linde-Zwirble W, et al. Association between positive airway pressure therapy adherence and health care resource utilization in patients with obstructive sleep apnea and type 2 diabetes in the United States. J Clin Sleep Med 2022. https://doi.org/10.5664/jcsm.10388.

14. Pépin JL, Baillieul S, Tamisier R. Reshaping sleep apnea care: time for value-based strategies. Ann Am Thorac Soc 2019;16(12):1501–3.

15. Estill J. Knowledge is the key to prevention: managing the silent epidemic of sleep apnoea. Lancet Reg Health Eur 2022;16:100377.

16. Kapur VK, Auckley DH, Chowdhuri S, et al. Clinical practice guideline for diagnostic testing for adult obstructive sleep apnea: an American Academy of sleep medicine clinical practice guideline. J Clin Sleep Med 2017;13(3):479–504.

17. Roeder M, Kohler M. It's time for multiple sleep night testing in OSA. Chest 2020;158(1):33–4.

18. Punjabi NM, Patil S, Crainiceanu C, et al. Variability and misclassification of sleep apnea severity based on multi-night testing. Chest 2020;158(1):365–73.

19. Roeder M, Bradicich M, Schwarz EI, et al. Night-to-night variability of respiratory events in obstructive sleep apnoea: a systematic review and meta-analysis. Thorax 2020;75(12):1095–102.

20. Chouraki A, Tournant J, Arnal P, et al. Objective multi-night sleep monitoring at home: variability of sleep parameters between nights and implications for the reliability of sleep assessment in clinical trials. Sleep 2022;zsac319. https://doi.org/10.1093/sleep/zsac319.

21. Lechat B, Naik G, Reynolds A, et al. Multinight prevalence, variability, and diagnostic misclassification of obstructive sleep apnea. Am J Respir Crit Care Med 2022;205(5):563–9.

22. Abreu A, Punjabi NM. How many nights are really needed to diagnose obstructive sleep apnea? Am J Respir Crit Care Med 2022;206(1):125–6.

23. Pépin JL, Letesson C, Le-Dong NN, et al. Assessment of mandibular movement monitoring with machine learning analysis for the diagnosis of obstructive sleep apnea. JAMA Netw Open 2020; 3(1):e1919657.

24. Le-Dong NN, Martinot JB, Coumans N, et al. Machine learning-based sleep staging in patients with sleep apnea using a single mandibular movement signal. Am J Respir Crit Care Med 2021;204(10): 1227–31.

25. Kelly JL, Ben Messaoud R, Joyeux-Faure M, et al. Diagnosis of sleep apnoea using a mandibular monitor and machine learning analysis: one-night agreement compared to in-home polysomnography. Front Neurosci 2022;16:726880.

26. Schnall RP, Sheffy JK, Penzel T. Peripheral arterial tonometry-PAT technology. Sleep Med Rev 2022; 61:101566.

27. Verhaert DVM, Betz K, Gawałko M, et al. A VIRTUAL Sleep Apnoea management pathway for the work-up of Atrial fibrillation patients in a digital Remote Infrastructure: virtual-SAFARI. Europace 2022; 24(4):565–75.

28. Simonds AK. How many more nights? Diagnosing and classifying obstructive sleep apnea using multi-night home studies. Am J Respir Crit Care Med 2022;205(5):491–2.

29. Lechat B, Catcheside P, Reynolds A, et al. Reply to Martinez-Garcia et al. and to Abreu and Punjabi. Am J Respir Crit Care Med 2022;206(1):126–9.

30. Lévy P, Tamisier R, Pépin JL. Assessment of sleep-disordered-breathing: quest for a metric or search for meaning? J Sleep Res 2020;29(4):e13143.

31. Linz D, Brooks AG, Elliott AD, et al. Variability of sleep apnea severity and risk of atrial fibrillation: the VARIOSA-AF study. JACC Clin Electrophysiol 2019;5(6):692–701.

32. Mazza A, Bendini MG, Bianchi V, et al. Association between device-detected sleep-disordered breathing and implantable defibrillator therapy in patients

with heart failure. JACC Clin Electrophysiol 2022; 8(10):1249–56.

33. Lechat B, Nguyen DP, Reynolds A, et al. Single night diagnosis of sleep apnea contributes to inconsistent cardiovascular outcome findings. Chest 2023. https://doi.org/10.1016/j.chest.2023.01.027. S0012-3692(23)00157-00165.

34. Lechat B, Scott H, Naik G, et al. New and emerging approaches to better define sleep disruption and its consequences. Front Neurosci 2021;15:751730.

35. Choo BP, Mok Y, Oh HC, et al. Benchmarking performance of an automatic polysomnography scoring system in a population with suspected sleep disorders. Front Neurol 2023;14:1123935.

36. Martinot JB, Le-Dong NN, Malhotra A, et al. Respiratory effort during sleep and prevalent hypertension in obstructive sleep apnoea. Eur Respir J 2022;2201486.

37. Iftikhar IH, Finch CE, Shah AS, et al. A meta-analysis of diagnostic test performance of peripheral arterial tonometry studies. J Clin Sleep Med 2022;18(4): 1093–102.

38. Pepin JL, Le-Dong NN, Cuthbert V, et al. Mandibular movements are a reliable noninvasive alternative to esophageal pressure for measuring respiratory effort in patients with sleep apnea syndrome. Nat Sci Sleep 2022;14:635–44.

39. Ioachimescu OC. On PAT, patterns and paths. Sleep 2022;45(5):zsac057.

40. Massie F, Mendes de Almeida D, Dreesen P, et al. An evaluation of the NightOwl home sleep apnea testing system. J Clin Sleep Med 2018;14(10): 1791–6.

41. Magalang UJ, Chen NH, Cistulli PA, et al. Agreement in the scoring of respiratory events and sleep among international sleep centers. Sleep 2013;36(4):591–6.

42. Fiorillo L, Puiatti A, Papandrea M, et al. Automated sleep scoring: a review of the latest approaches. Sleep Med Rev 2019;48:101204.

43. Berger M, Vakulin A, Hirotsu C, et al. Association between sleep microstructure and incident hypertension in a population-based sample: the HypnoLaus study. J Am Heart Assoc 2022;11(14):e025828.

44. Vollmer S, Mateen BA, Bohner G, et al. Machine learning and artificial intelligence research for patient benefit: 20 critical questions on transparency, replicability, ethics, and effectiveness. BMJ 2020; 368:l6927.

45. Plana D, Shung DL, Grimshaw AA, et al. Randomized clinical trials of machine learning interventions in health care: a systematic review. JAMA Netw Open 2022;5(9):e2233946.

46. Baumert M, Cowie MR, Redline S, et al. Sleep characterization with smart wearable devices: a call for standardization and consensus recommendations. Sleep 2022;45(12):zsac183.

47. An J, Glick HA, Sawyer AM, et al. Association between positive airway pressure adherence and healthcare costs among individuals with obstructive sleep apnea. Chest 2023. https://doi.org/10.1016/j. chest.2023.01.025. S0012-3692(23)00132-00140.

Consumer Wearable Sleep Trackers
Are They Ready for Clinical Use?

Ambrose A. Chiang, MD, FCCP, FAASM[a,b,c,]*,
Seema Khosla, MD, FCCP, FAASM[d]

KEYWORDS

- Wearable • Consumer sleep technology • Photoplethysmography • Actigraphy • Sleep stage
- Sleep apnea • Pulse oximetry • Heart rate variability

KEY POINTS

- Sleep continues to gain more recognition among the general public. Consequently, the self-monitoring of sleep has become a familiar refrain. Patients routinely gauge the quality of their sleep based on wearable-provided metrics, which may have variable clinical relevance.
- Current technologies are more sophisticated, with high-performance miniaturized electronic sensors and rapid advancements in software development. This continues to blur the boundaries between medical-grade and consumer-grade wearable devices.
- Consumer wearable sleep trackers (CWSTs) data have spilled into routine sleep clinic visits. Sleep clinicians must understand their performance and navigate this new terrain, often relying on clinical instinct, familiarity with technology, and personal comfort, in order to integrate this patient-generated healthcare data into a clinical visit, understanding that these data can vary significantly depending upon the technology and the clinical presentation.
- We believe that CWST devices should remain in the general wellness domain. In specific scenarios where clinicians and researchers use CWSTs, the CWSTs with the best performance should be used. The interpretation of wearable-generated sleep data must remain within the confines of a comprehensive sleep assessment.
- In addition to current concerns, future challenges require collaboration between clinicians, manufacturers, researchers, professional societies, and regulatory agencies. A framework will need to be developed and implemented, recognizing the rapid advancement of technology and the slow pace of adoption and consensus among these stakeholders.

INTRODUCTION

Sleep medicine is experiencing a moment. The 2017 Nobel Prize was awarded to circadian rhythm researchers for their discoveries of molecular mechanisms controlling the circadian rhythm.[1] The media attention around sleep is high, and there is compelling data to support sleep as the third pillar of health, along with nutrition and exercise.[2] Because interest in improving sleep continues, consumers are searching for ways to improve their sleep.

Wearable sensor technology has grown and advanced from crude activity and sleep tracking to more granular sleep health and physiological assessment.[3–12] The incorporation of photoplethysmography (PPG) into accelerometry, the application of artificial intelligence/machine learning/deep learning (AI/ML/DL) algorithms, and the addition of

[a] Division of Sleep Medicine, Louis Stokes Cleveland VA Medical Center, 10701 East Blvd, Suite 2B-129, Cleveland, OH 44106, USA; [b] Division of Pulmonary, Critical Care, and Sleep Medicine, University Hospitals Cleveland Medical Center, Cleveland, OH, USA; [c] Department of Medicine, Case Western Reserve University, Cleveland, OH, USA; [d] North Dakota Center for Sleep, 1531 32nd Avenue S Ste 103, Fargo, ND 58103, USA
* Corresponding author.
E-mail address: Ambrose.chiang@va.gov

Sleep Med Clin 18 (2023) 311–330
https://doi.org/10.1016/j.jsmc.2023.05.005
1556-407X/23/Published by Elsevier Inc.

pulse oximetry and heart rate variability (HRV) data to the consumer wearable sleep trackers (CWST) allow for potential broader consumer and clinical utility.[4,7,13,14] However, given the lack of regulatory oversight and third-party performance assessment, the accuracy of the functionalities of most CWSTs on the market remains questionable.[9]

Overall, industry claims are challenging to decipher. Although the declarative statements by CWSTs are impressive, it can be difficult to determine their clinical usefulness. Some of this apprehension relates to the opacity of the CWST algorithms.[14] Moreover, some industry terms for categorizing sleep are not precisely defined and are unfamiliar to clinicians. For instance, what exactly does a "sleep score" represent? Is it based on sleep duration, sleep efficiency, sleep stage percentage, awakenings, pulse rate variability (PRV), oxygen saturation, or some combination?[15–17] Manufacturers often have their own definitions or terms that are neither explicitly defined nor standardized. Most importantly, uncertainties may relate to the accuracy of the collected data and how these data compare to PSG, our "gold standard."[18] Ultimately, clinicians need assurance that the CWST data are reasonably accurate, at least for healthy individuals.

This article does not intend to cover every smartwatch, wristband, or ring comprehensively. Several review articles have been published in Sleep Medicine Clinics in the past 2 years.[10–12,19–21] We aim to add new information to the existing literature and review recent publications on PPG/accelerometry-based CWST devices in an attempt to answer a fundamental question, "Are consumer sleep trackers ready for clinical use?" Consequently, medical-grade wearables, smartphone applications, nearables, and under-the-bed devices are beyond the scope of this article.

In this review, we discuss the evolving sophistication of CWSTs and examine the continuum from consumer-grade to medical-grade devices. We explore the functionalities generated by these devices and their use in healthy individuals versus those with underlying sleep disorders. We also investigate how clinicians must decide if the CWST data have value and, if so, how to incorporate the available patient-generated health data into a patient care plan in different clinical scenarios. A discussion of suggested clinical use is undertaken with the understanding that because these standards are created, the technology continues to evolve. As such, recommendations for appropriate use will always lag behind. Lastly, we discussed the current issues and future challenges. It should also be noted that mentioning specific CWSTs in this review does not imply the endorsement of any products by the authors.

MEDICAL-GRADE VERSUS CONSUMER-GRADE WEARABLES

Historically, one would consider a wearable device medical-grade when the device is cleared by the U.S. Food & Drug Administration (FDA) as a class II device either through the 510(k) process or through the de novo pathway.[6] **Table 1** summarizes the differences between medical-grade and consumer-grade wearables.

Despite these differences, the boundaries between medical and consumer-grade wearable devices have become increasingly blurred in recent years because of rapid wearable technological advancement and performance improvement.[22] Recent evidence suggests that some CWSTs perform about as well as medical-grade actigraphy in estimating sleep–wake in healthy volunteers.[23,24] Another contributing factor to this blurriness is that FDA clearance may be granted for only some functionalities but not all the claimed ones. For example, the FDA has cleared several CWSTs for ECG and irregular rhythm notification functions. Yet, the pulse oximetry function of the same devices may not be cleared.[25,26] Hence, a device may be "partially" medical-grade.

Another point worth noting is the difference between FDA registration and FDA clearance.[6] An FDA-registered device is only recognized by the FDA for general wellness or sports use and does not denote FDA clearance.[27] Consequently, it is appropriate for an FDA-registered CWST to explore, track, and record sleep as part of a healthy lifestyle, but unfitting for the device to diagnose or treat a disease/condition. It has been the position of the AASM that sleep technologies must be FDA-cleared and rigorously tested against gold standards if intended to render a diagnosis and/or treatment.[18]

RECENT CONSUMER WEARABLE SLEEP TRACKER TECHNOLOGICAL ADVANCES
Advances in Hardware: The Miniaturization of Electronic Sensors

In addition to the integration of PPG with accelerometry, modern wearable technology has been made possible by high-performance miniaturized electronic sensors and advancements in AI/ML/DL algorithms.[3,7,28,29] Multi-sensor CWSTs typically assess and track sleep using the physiological data collected from the PPG and 3-axis accelerometer. In some CWSTs, a gyroscope (which measures rotation and orientation) and temperature sensors are also employed, such as in the Oura ring. The emerging miniaturized "earable" technology has certain technological and

Table 1
Consumer-grade versus medical-grade wearables

	Consumer-Grade Wearables	Medical-Grade Wearables
Alternative names	Commercial-grade	Clinical-grade, research-grade, or scientific-grade
FDA clearance status	Not cleared	Cleared by the FDA for at least one functionality[a]
FDA oversight/regulation	No	Yes
Targeted populations	Healthy individuals	Patients with sleep disturbances
Targeted use	General wellness or sports use	Clinical use for detection or follow-up of sleep disorders
Performance supported by research	Most have no or limited research	Better supported by the literature
Research in patients with sleep disorders	Limited	More common
Utilization by clinicians	Uncommonly used	Varies
Prescription needed	No	Yes
Costs	Varies	Typically more expensive than consumer devices
Purchase	Through retailers or online vendors	Through distributors or retailers

Abbreviation: FDA, U.S. Food & Drug Administration.
　[a] FDA clearance may be granted only for certain functionalities and not for all claimed functionalities.

physiological advantages.[29] **Table 2** shows the advantages and disadvantages of various types of CWSTs.

Advances in Software: The Incorporation of Artificial Intelligence/Machine Learning/Deep Learning Algorithms

Another essential advancement in wearable technology is the rapid evolution and broad application of AI/ML/DL technologies, particularly in DL neural networks.[14,28,29,31] Conventional rule-based algorithms are developed based on the features/criteria delineated by humans and were employed in actigraphy and older-generation wearable devices.[32–34] As rule-based algorithms are constructed from simple "if-then" commands based on already known knowledge, the performance of rule-based algorithms may be limited when there are a vast number of intertwined or unrecognized variables. Conversely, a DL neural network, a complex mathematical system fed with a large set of raw data to develop its own multi-layer representations, can potentially identify subtle features from the input signals beyond what the naked eye can identify and handle complex and intricate relationships.[35] With more datasets collected and fed for DL algorithm retraining over time, the extracted features can be optimized for

improved performance. Recent studies have demonstrated that AI/ML/DL algorithms using PPG signals can enable sleep stage classification, OSA detection, and apnea severity categorization.[36–38] **Table 3** illustrates the fundamental differences between traditional rule-based and DL algorithms.

CONSUMER WEARABLE SLEEP TRACKER SLEEP-RELATED FUNCTIONALITIES
The Performance of Consumer Wearable Sleep Trackers in Assessing Sleep in Healthy Individuals

The performance of consumer wearable sleep trackers in estimating sleep–wake outcomes in healthy individuals
It is widely acknowledged that medical-grade actigraphy devices tend to overestimate sleep and underestimate wakefulness.[39–41] These devices typically have a high sensitivity (0.91–0.96) in detecting sleep and a low-to-medium specificity (0.34–0.63) in detecting wakefulness. Earlier CWST performance evaluation studies using Jawbone UP, the original Fitbit tracker, and Fitbit Charge HR in adolescents and adults showed similar results with high sensitivity (0.97–0.98) and low specificity (0.20–0.42).[42–44] More recent studies using wrist-worn devices (Fitbit Surge,

Table 2
Comparison between various types of consumer wearable sleep trackers

	Wrist-Worn Devices	Rings	Earables[30]
Sensor location	• Back of the wrist	• Proximal phalanx of fingers	• External ear canal
Potential Advantages	• Sensors embedded in watches or wristbands • May be used 24/7	• Sensors embedded in specially designed rings • May have better contact than wrist-worn devices • Hair is typically not an issue • May be used 24/7	• Can potentially incorporate ear-EEG • Less affected by movement during the daytime • Less external electrical noise • PPG signal is resistant to blood volume changes during hypothermia • More accurate core body temperature measurement
Potential Disadvantages	• Less-than-ideal PPG signals because of low vascularity at the back of the wrist, poor contact, motion artifacts, sweats, tattoos, and hairs • Discomfort if too tight	• Signal quality may be sensitive to the rotation of the ring • Limited battery power	• Ear wax, chewing, and talking may affect signals • Potential discomfort in sleep when sleeping sideways • Limited battery power

Abbreviations: EEG, electroencephalogram; PPG, photoplethysmography.

Charge 2, Alta HR, and Apple Watch) demonstrated high sensitivity (0.93–0.98) and improved specificity (0.51–0.69).[45–49] Two studies that assessed the Oura ring showed a sensitivity of 0.96 and a specificity of 0.41 to 0.48.[49,50] Most recently, Miller and colleagues examined the performance of 6 wearable devices (Apple Watch Series 6, Garmin Forerunner 245 Music, Polar Vantage V, Oura ring Generation 2, WHOOP 3.0, and Somfit, which is a forehead patch PPG-based device) in 53 healthy young adults.[51] Sleep–wake analysis showed a sensitivity of 0.90 to 0.97 and

Table 3
Rule-based versus deep learning algorithm

	Rule-Based Algorithm	Deep Learning Algorithm
Instructions	• Constructed by humans	• Constructed by the DL algorithm (with human inputs)
Structure	• Decision tree	• Varied based on the DL model used
Potential Advantages	• Logical and unambiguous • Easy to understand (if "a", then "b")	• Not limited by human knowledge • Can potentially identify subtle features from the input signals beyond what the naked eye can discern • Can better assess complex data and intricate relationships • Algorithms are easier to retrain and fine-tune when more datasets are available
Potential Disadvantages	• Limited by human knowledge • May not be able to effectively handle complex relationships	• "Black box" • Humans may not fully understand how the algorithms work exactly

Abbreviation: DL, deep learning.

a specificity of 0.26 to 0.57. Cohen's Kappa varied from 0.30 to 0.51, and total sleep time (TST) bias varied from −5.5 to 43.8 min with a wide SD of 36.3 to 45.3 min.

Chinoy and colleagues conducted a study comparing multiple consumer sleep technologies, including 4 CWST devices (Fatigue Science Readiband, Fitbit Alta HR, Garmin Fenix 5S, Garmin Vivosmart 3), to in-lab PSG along with Actiwatch 2 in 34 healthy young adults.[23] These 4 CWST devices showed high sensitivity in detecting sleep but low specificity in detecting wake (0.18–0.54). Notably, some devices demonstrated comparable or even superior performance to the Actiwatch (specificity: Fitbit Alta HR 0.54 vs Actiwatch 0.39). This implies some CWST devices can be potential alternatives to actigraphy, at least for sleep–wake outcomes in healthy young individuals. A follow-up trial by the same group compared the performance of 4 CWST devices (Fatigue Science Readiband, Fitbit Inspire HR, Oura Ring Generation 2, and Polar Vantage V Titan) to the Actiwatch 2 under unrestricted natural home sleep conditions against the research version Dreem 2 mobile EEG headband in 21 healthy young adults for 7 nights.[24] CWST sleep–wake outcomes were generally more accurate on nights with more consolidated sleep. The specificity for wake ranged from 0.35 to 0.45, equivalent to or higher than Actiwatch 2 specificity (0.35). The authors concluded that most tested CWST devices compared favorably to actigraphy in wake detection.

The performance of consumer wearable sleep trackers in classifying sleep stages in healthy individuals

Beatties and colleagues evaluated the accuracy of sleep stage classification using the Fitbit Surge in 60 healthy adult participants. The authors demonstrated an epoch-by-epoch (EBE) agreement of 69%, 62%, and 72% in detecting light (N1 + N2), deep (N3), and REM sleep, respectively.[45] The overall EBE accuracy was 69%, and Cohen's kappa was 0.52. Miller and colleagues showed similar results by assessing 12 healthy young adults using the WHOOP strap in a 10 day, lab-based protocol. Their overall EBE agreement was 64%, with a multi-stage agreement of 62%, 68%, and 70% in detecting light, deep, and REM sleep.[49] In a study by de Zambotti and colleagues, the Fitbit Charge 2 was assessed in 44 healthy adults, which showed an accuracy of 81%, 49%, and 74% in detecting light, deep, and REM sleep, respectively.[46] de Zambotti and colleagues also evaluated the performance of the Oura ring against PSG in 41 healthy adolescents and young adults. Oura ring demonstrated an EBE agreement of 65%, 51%, and 61% in detecting light, deep, and REM sleep, respectively.[50]

In the Miller study with 6 wearable devices, the EBE multi-stage analysis showed an agreement of 44% to 68%, 28% to 65%, and 49% to 66% in detecting light, deep, and REM sleep, respectively.[51] The overall agreement varied from 50% to 65%. In the 2021 Chinoy study, 1 Fitbit and 2 Garmin devices achieved an EBE sleep stage agreement of 68% to 76%, 53% to 56%, and 50% to 69% in detecting light, deep, and REM sleep, respectively.[23] In the 2022 Chinoy study in unrestricted natural home environments, the EBE sleep stage performance of the 4 CWSTs tested also varied significantly (59%–71%, 51%–72%, and 36%–47% in detecting light, deep, and REM sleep, respectively).[24] Chinoy and colleagues concluded that CWSTs may be better reserved for tracking sleep–wake outcomes than discerning sleep stages, given the substantial performance variability in classifying sleep stages.

The Performance of Consumer Wearable Sleep Trackers in Assessing Sleep–Wake in Patients with Sleep Disorders

CWST performance trials for sleep assessment were mostly performed in young, healthy populations but scarcely in those with sleep disturbances. Because CWSTs tend to overestimate sleep and underestimate wake, their performance would likely be poorer in those with fragmented sleep and frequent sleep–wake or sleep stage transitions.[48] For this reason, performance studies in subjects with disturbed sleep are essential before we can confidently interpret the results in this population.

The performance of consumer wearable sleep trackers in patients with insomnia

Kang and colleagues were the first to assess the performance of CWST in patients with insomnia.[52] The authors compared Actiwatch 2 and Fitbit Flex, an earlier Fitbit model without PPG, to unattended portable PSG in 33 adult patients with insomnia and 17 good sleepers. The Fitbit Flex EBE specificity was low in the good-sleeper (0.36) and insomnia groups (0.36). Actiwatch 2, on the other hand, had a higher specificity of 0.45 in the insomnia group and 0.61 in good sleepers. Overall, the performance of the Fitbit Flex was inferior to that of the Actiwatch 2.

Khawaja and colleagues assessed the performance of the Fitbit Alta HR and Actiwatch Spectrum Pro against in-lab PSG in 42 patients diagnosed with chronic insomnia.[53] Actiwatch and Fitbit Alta HR demonstrated low specificity (0.39 and 0.45, respectively; $P = .037$). Both significantly overestimated TST (Fitbit 53.3 min and Actiwatch 64.2 min) and underestimated wake. The authors concluded that the Fitbit Alta HR was better than the Actiwatch at detecting wakefulness in patients with insomnia. More recently, Dong assessed the performance of Fitbit Charge 4 and Actiwatch Spectrum Pro against PSG in 37 Chinese patients with chronic insomnia.[54] Fitbit had significantly better specificity (0.62) in detecting wake than Actiwatch (0.36), which added to the existing evidence that certain CWSTs can outperform medical-grade actigraphy in detecting wake in patients with chronic insomnia. In this study, Fitbit Charge 4 demonstrated no significant bias in assessing TST and REM sleep but notably underestimated deep sleep while remarkably overestimating light sleep.

The performance of consumer wearable sleep trackers in patients suspected of OSA

Toon and colleagues first compared Jawbone UP and Actiwatch 2 to in-lab PSG in 78 children and adolescents with suspected OSA.[55] Jawbone UP showed good sensitivity (0.92) and medium specificity (0.66) with an overestimation of TST by 9 min (vs 17 min in Actiwatch 2). The authors concluded that Jawbone UP was comparable to Actiwatch 2 in children and adolescents suspected of sleep apnea. In contrast, the study results of CWSTs in adults suspected of OSA were not as encouraging. Gruwez and colleagues evaluated the performance of Withings Pulse O2 and Jawbone Up against in-lab PSG in 36 adults suspected of OSA.[56] The authors found poor validity for all parameters with both devices and concluded that the performance of these 2 devices was limited in this patient population. Moreno-Pino et al. assessed the Fitbit Charge 2 and the Fitbit Alta HR against PSG in 65 participants.[57] Fitbit devices overestimated TST by 59.8 min and underestimated WASO by 36.1 min. The overall specificity for wake was low (0.44), and the authors concluded that these Fitbit devices do not have sufficient accuracy for clinical use in adults suspected of OSA.

The performance of consumer wearable sleep trackers in patients suspected of central disorders of hypersomnolence

In the 2018 AASM actigraphy Clinical Practice guideline, the AASM Task Force suggested that actigraphy may be used for monitoring TST for 7 to 14 days before PSG/MSLT but is not intended to replace PSG.[58] Cook and colleagues evaluated Jawbone UP3 in 43 patients with suspected central disorders of hypersomnolence who underwent concurrent PSG/MSLT and Actiwatch 2.[59] Jawbone demonstrated a significant overestimation of TST (39.6 min) relative to PSG but performed comparably to Actiwatch. Its ability to distinguish light, deep, and REM sleep was poor. The authors concluded that Jawbone UP3 cannot be used as a diagnostic surrogate for PSG or MSLT in assessing patients with suspected central disorders of hypersomnolence.

CONSUMER WEARABLE SLEEP TRACKER PULSE OXIMETRY
Finger pulse oximetry versus consumer wearable sleep tracker's pulse oximetry

Commercial low-cost finger pulse oximeters have emerged as a widely used tool for spot-checking home oxygen saturation (SpO2) for patients with cardiopulmonary disorders. However, the performance of most over-the-counter finger pulse oximeters has not been validated.[60] Some finger pulse oximeters provide overnight SpO2 monitoring, but they can easily dislodge in sleep. In contrast, most CWSTs can be worn firmly on the wrist or finger.[61] However, it is worth noting that, unlike finger pulse oximeters that measure SpO2 from fingertips where vascularity is rich, wrist-worn CWSTs measure SpO2 from the back of the wrists where vascularity is poor. In addition, wrist-worn CWSTs are subject to signal noise because of poor contact, sweat, hair, tattoos, or skin thickness, making accurate SpO2 measurements challenging in some cases (see **Table 1**).[62]

The performance of a consumer wearable sleep tracker pulse oximetry for SpO2 measurement

During the COVID-19 pandemic, SpO2 measurement demands increased sharply, and many manufacturers swiftly incorporated SpO2 measurement into their CWSTs. Although CWST pulse oximetry is sometimes used for SpO2 on-demand spot checks (as in the Apple Watch Series 6), most CWSTs provide nocturnal SpO2 values and display SpO2 tracing through downloaded apps.[63,64] Newer Fitbit wrist-worn devices provide average overnight SpO2 with trend display through Fitbit apps.[64]

It is pertinent to understand that CWSTs must meet the 2013 FDA pulse oximeter 510(k) submission guidance for the pulse oximetry functionality to be cleared by the FDA.[65] The FDA requires that in vivo testing with arterial catheterization and blood sampling be performed under lab conditions with various FiO_2 to achieve a SpO2 of 70% to 100%. At least 200 paired sample data points from 10 or more healthy subjects that vary in age, gender, and skin pigmentation must be included. The 2013 FDA Guidance requires a root-mean-square difference (A_{rms}) of $\leq 3.0\%$ for transmittance and 3.5% for reflectance pulse oximetry.[65] The FDA also recommended that every premarket clinical study submitted should have participants with a range of skin pigmentations, including at least 2 darkly pigmented participants or 15% of the participant pool, whichever is greater.[65]

As of this writing, Withings ScanWatch is the only CWST with FDA-cleared pulse oximetry.[66] No others, including the Apple Watch, Fitbit, and Oura ring, have FDA clearance for pulse oximetry functionality. Kirszenblat and colleagues evaluated the performance accuracy of the Withings ScanWatch SpO2 against SaO2 in 14 healthy young adults (3/14 with dark skin tone) in a hypoxia laboratory.[61] The authors found that the Withings ScanWatch can measure SpO2 with adequate accuracy at a medical-grade level ($A_{rms} \leq 3.0\%$.). Notably, its accuracy in older adults, patients with cardiopulmonary disorders, or real-life situations has not been established.

Pipek compared the Apple Watch Series 6 to 2 "commercial" finger pulse oximeters in 100 patients with COPD and interstitial lung disease for spot checks in a resting state at a pulmonary clinic and reported a positive correlation in SpO2 measurements.[67] Spaccarotella and colleagues compared the Apple Watch Series 6 to the Nellcor pulse oximeter, an FDA-cleared medical-grade pulse oximeter, in 257 Caucasian participants, with the majority having cardiovascular or pulmonary disorders.[68] The authors showed that the Apple Watch Series 6 SpO2 measurement was strongly correlated with the Nellcor SpO2. Of note, both studies were performed in clinics with the assistance of trained staff following stringent protocols but not in an unrestricted casual home setting, and the gold standard SaO2 was not measured. Apple recently published online the performance of the Apple Watch Blood Oxygen app by comparing its SpO2 to SaO2 in 50 healthy adults, including 8 individuals with dark skin tones.[69] The 70% to 100% A_{rms} was 2.18% SpO2 in the final 24-subject validation set.

The Performance of Consumer Wearable Sleep Tracker Pulse Oximetry for Oxygen Desaturation Index

Some CWSTs report Oxygen Desaturation Index (ODI) and SpO2 nadir, as in the case of Circul/Circul+, an FDA-registered device.[70] ODI has been controversial as an Apnea-Hypopnea Index (AHI) predictor because of large discrepancies in

sensitivities (32%–99%) and specificities (48%–98%) at various AHI cutoffs.[71] Zhao recently evaluated the accuracy of Circul-ODI3% in 207 Chinese subjects suspected of OSA.[72] A significant difference between PSG-ODI and Circul-ODI (25.3 vs 22.2 events/h, respectively, $P < .0001$) was observed. Using Circul-ODI of 5 to predict PSG-AHI of 5, Circul had an accuracy, sensitivity, and specificity of 0.86, 0.87, and 0.83, respectively. Using a Circul-ODI cutoff of 15 events/h, Circul had an accuracy, sensitivity, and specificity of 0.76, 0.66, and 0.96, respectively. It remains unclear if the results can be generalized to those with a higher BMI or populations with darker skin tones. Notably, using ODI to predict, screen, or diagnose OSA is beyond the FDA's general wellness category for CWST and cannot be endorsed.

The Performance of the Consumer Wearable Sleep Tracker Apnea-Hypopnea Index

Wearable devices that provide AHI for OSA detection require FDA clearance. Hence, CWSTs rarely provide AHI. Still, some manufacturers report AHI through smartphone apps. For instance, Go2sleep (SLEEPON, USA) reports AHI despite the lack of published performance evaluation studies or FDA clearance.[73] Although the SLEEPON website does provide patient education information concerning how AHI is calculated and how OSA severity is defined, SLEEPON offers no recommendations concerning how to use this information or when customers should seek medical attention.[74]

The influence of darker skin tones on the accuracy of pulse oximetry

Another recent concern is the accuracy of pulse oximetry in populations with darker skin tones. Sjoding retrospectively studied adult inpatients in 2 large cohorts and showed that black patients had nearly three times the frequency of occult hypoxemia (defined as SaO2 of <88% despite SpO2 of 92%–96% on finger pulse oximetry) that was not detected by finger pulse oximetry in white patients.[75] The authors suggested that there is "racial bias" and that reliance on pulse oximetry SpO2 measurement for clinical decisions may put black patients at increased risk for hypoxemia. In response to this concern, the FDA issued a safety communication about pulse oximeter accuracy and limitations in 2021.[76] The FDA emphasized the following points.

- The SpO2 reading should always be considered an "estimate" of SaO2, and the real-world accuracy may differ from the lab setting.

- Significant SpO2 variation may exist even in FDA-cleared pulse oximeters. The typical accuracy (reported as A_{rms}) of recently FDA-cleared pulse oximeters is within 2% to 3% of SaO2. If an FDA-cleared pulse oximeter reads 90%, the true SaO2 is generally between 86% and 94%.
- Pulse oximeter accuracy is highest at 90% to 100%, intermediate at 80% to 90%, and lowest below 80%.
- The accuracy differences in pulse oximeters between dark and light skin pigmentation are typically small at saturations $\geq$ 80% and greater when saturations are less than 80%.

In November 2022, the FDA published an executive summary reviewing pulse oximeters and factors that may impact their accuracy.[77] FDA conducted a PubMed search using the strategy "pulse oxim* AND (race OR racial OR pigment)" and published a systematic literature review of the real-world performance of pulse oximeters, including 3 relevant systemic reviews published in 2022 (Section VIII).[78–80] It was concluded that mounting evidence suggests the performance of pulse oximeters can be affected by skin pigmentation. Currently, little is known about the performance of CWST pulse oximetry in patients with darker skin tones. Further research in this area is warranted.

CONSUMER WEARABLE SLEEP TRACKER PULSE RATE VARIABILITY
Consumer wearable sleep tracker pulse rate variability versus ECG heart rate variability

Pulse rate variability (often regarded as HRV) is another common CWST feature. HRV is calculated from the R–R intervals of the QRS complex extracted from the ECG, which allows indirect, noninvasive measurement of autonomic nervous system (ANS) activities. HRV varies with age, gender, physical fitness, and overall health, including mental and physical conditions.[81,82] The time-domain and frequency-domain HRV parameters can be derived to represent sympathetic, parasympathetic, or global ANS activities (**Table 4**).[81–85] HRV is being increasingly applied in various medical fields, and many studies have demonstrated the association of low HRV with a higher risk of all-cause death and cardiovascular events.[86] Low HRV is also associated with sleep and psychiatric disorders, such as OSA, insomnia, depression, anxiety, and PTSD, and can be potentially used as a biomarker for increased suicidality.[87–93]

In contrast, PPG-based PRV in CWST is derived from PPG peak-to-peak intervals and has often been used as a surrogate of HRV.[95,96] CWST PRV is commonly utilized for general fitness, physical training balance, and assessment of psychological stress.[97] However, it is crucial to recognize that the relationship between HRV and PRV is not fully understood and may not be as straightforward as we think.[96] Pinheiro and colleagues found that PRV metrics can be used as an alternative for HRV analysis in healthy subjects with good correlations, for time-domain and frequency-domain features. Conversely, in subjects with cardiovascular disorders, time-domain and, most importantly, frequency-domain metrics should be used with caution.[98] Mejia-Mejia et al. recently suggested that although PRV may be a reasonable proxy of HRV in young, healthy subjects in the supine, controlled, resting state, it should not be considered a valid HRV surrogate in all scenarios because PRV might be influenced by technical and physiological factors, particularly during nonstationary conditions or in unhealthy subjects.[96]

How pulse rate variability is measured by consumer wearable sleep trackers?

HRV is typically measured based on 5 min data or as a 24 h average. Still, it can also be calculated as an average of sleep.[81,83,85] Sleep is, theoretically, an ideal time for measurement of parasympathetic activities in individuals without sleep disorders because heart rate is mainly under parasympathetic control during supine rest, and there are fewer stressors or motion artifacts in sleep.[83] Root mean squares of successive RR interval differences (RMSSD), the primary time-domain PRV metric reflecting parasympathetic activity, is the most commonly used CWST PRV parameter. Many CWSTs, such as Fitbit, WHOOP, and Oura ring, measure PRV primarily during a full night's sleep. For instance, Oura ring measures PRV in sleep by calculating the mean of all 5 min RMSSD samples.[99] Other CWSTs, such as Apple and Samsung watches, measure on-demand HRV over 3 to 5 minutes during the day, often recommending measuring immediately upon awakening.[100,101]

The performance of consumer wearable sleep tracker pulse rate variability

Few studies have examined the correlation between the CWST PRV and ECG HRV metrics, and even fewer have investigated PRV during sleep.[51,102] Stone and colleagues recently assessed the resting-state RMSSD in 4 devices, including the Oura ring Gen 2, by comparing them against ECG for 3 or 5 min in an upright, seated position with a total of 148 trials in 5 healthy

Table 4
Commonly used time-domain and frequency-domain heart rate variability parameters

HRV parameters[81]	Physiology	Significance
Time-domain		
SDNN (ms)	Global autonomic regulation; SNS and PNS activities	SDNN reflects total HRV, predicts morbidity and mortality, and is considered the gold standard for medical stratification of cardiac risk when recorded over a 24 h period
RMSSD (ms)	PNS activity	The primary HRV metric used by CWSTs; correlates with HF power and PNN50
PNN50 (%)	PNS activity	Correlates with HF power and RMSSD
Frequency-domain		
HF Power (0.15–0.40 Hz)	PNS activity	Also called the respiratory band; corresponds to HR variations related to the respiratory cycle; an erratic rhythm can exaggerate HF power
LF Power (0.04–0.15 Hz)	SNS, PNS, baroreflex activities	LF power is not modulated only by SNS. The SNS contribution to LF power varies profoundly with testing conditions.
VLF Power (0.01–0.04 Hz)	Renin–angiotensin system, PNS activity	VLF power can be blocked by ACE inhibitors and atropine but not by beta-blockers; exaggerated by SDB
LF/HF ratio	Sympathovagal balance?	The relationship between PNS and SNS activities is nonlinear and nonreciprocal. The hypothesis that the LF/HF ratio can be used to quantify sympathovagal balance has been challenged.[94]

Abbreviations: CWST, consumer wearable sleep tracker; HF, high frequency; HRV, heart rate variability; LF, low frequency; PNN50, percentage of successive RR intervals that differ by more than 50 ms; PNS, parasympathetic nervous system; RMSSD, root mean square of successive RR interval differences; SDB, sleep-disordered breathing; SDNN, standard deviation of NN intervals; SNS, sympathetic nervous system; VLF, very low frequency.

young adults.[98] The concordance correlation coefficient was 0.91. Miller and colleagues assessed the validity of RMSSD in 6 CWST devices against ECG during or just before nighttime sleep in 53 healthy young adults.[51] The authors found PRV validity varied with devices, and the better-performing ones appeared to provide valid measurements in healthy young adults. Lam and colleagues compared Microsoft Band 2 PRV with portable ECG HRV during unsupervised free-living conditions, including sleep, in 10 healthy adults and concluded that PRV was a poor surrogate for HRV under free-living conditions.[103]

It is also worth mentioning that the HRV-PRV difference may increase with OSA and vascular aging.[96,104] Khandoker investigated the correlation between PRV and HRV in 29 healthy subjects during normal breathing and 22 patients with OSA during OSA events.[104] PRV provides accurate PRV to measure HRV under normal breathing in sleep but does not precisely reflect HRV in OSA. Significant PRV-HRV differences were noted in SDNN, RMSSD, HF power, and LF/HF during OSA events. In sum, the accuracy of CWST PRV metrics needs further evaluation in sleep, particularly in elderly populations and those with sleep apnea or cardiovascular disorders. Because some PRV metrics may be more affected than others by disease conditions, finding the appropriate PRV parameters to use would be critical.[105]

Factors that may affect consumer wearable sleep tracker pulse rate and pulse rate variability

Although CWSTs can detect pulse rate with acceptable accuracy in healthy individuals, some factors, such as darker skin tones, tattoos, hair, sweat, a high BMI, and skin thickness, may influence PR accuracy, particularly in wrist-worn devices.[106–108] Unlike medical-grade PPG-based devices (typically using red and infrared LED lights), most CWSTs use green light, with which PR may be affected by darker skin tones (Table 5).[62,106,107] Notably, not all studies showed that darker skin tone causes PR inaccuracy.[108] Bent investigated the sources of CWST PR inaccuracy by studying 53 adults of various skin tones. They found no statistically significant difference in accuracy across skin tones but noted significant differences between devices in responding to changes in activity.[108] To improve this potential deficiency, several CWST manufacturers have recently added red/infrared light sensors.[106]

CLINICAL SCENARIOS IN WHICH WEARABLES MAY BE USED

In an effort to delineate clinical scenarios where wearable technologies may be utilized, we followed a continuum of use cases and proposed an algorithm to incorporate the use of wearable devices into a clinical visit, from healthy users for general wellness purposes to patients with sleep disorders and the use of medical-grade wearables (Fig. 1).

Scenario #1: Healthy individuals using CWSTs for sleep tracking

This scenario is typically consumer-initiated without clinician input. Users examine their sleep using wearable technology—either primarily because of an interest in their sleep or secondarily by reviewing wearable sleep data for a device that was purchased for a non-sleep reason. This scenario is for general wellness and is consistent with the FDA's recommendation.[27] A legitimate question is whether wearing CWST changes sleep quality or quantity. Berryhill and colleagues recently studied the impact of CWST (WHOOP strap 2.0) on perceived sleep quality using the sleep disturbance short-form questionnaire of the Patient-Reported Outcomes Measurement Information System (PROMIS) in 32 young, healthy participants in a 14-day randomized crossover study.[109] The authors found CWST improved nighttime sleep quality after adjusting for age, sex, baseline, and order effect. The mean reduction in the PROMIS sleep disturbance score was 1.69, which is small but statistically significant. However, the underlying mechanisms for the observed improvement are not exactly clear, and the long-term effects of CWSTs on sleep remain unanswered.[109,110]

Scenario #2: Patients with sleep disorders or symptoms using CWSTs for sleep tracking without clinicians' assistance

Scenario #2 is also consumer-initiated; however, the impetus to examine their sleep is dissatisfaction with their sleep. They may have an underlying sleep disorder, such as insomnia or OSA. Typically, these consumers not only track their sleep but also self-interpret the data and make adjustments based on the results. This group does not seek medical attention but prefers using CWST to improve their sleep. Notably, this scenario is no longer for general wellness but for self-treatment of sleep disorders, thus being inconsistent with the FDA's recommendation. This situation may be the most worrisome of all

Table 5
Comparison between green and red/infrared lights in consumer wearable sleep trackers[62]

	Green Light	Red and Infrared Light
Wavelengths	Shorter (490–570 nm)	Longer (620 nm to 1 mm)
Device type	Most CWSTs	Medical-grade devices and some CWSTs
Primary metric measured	Pulse rate	SpO2
Signal-to-noise ratio	Better	Poorer
Motion artifacts	Less susceptible	More susceptible
Skin absorption/penetration	More absorption, shallower penetration	Less absorption, deeper penetration
Affected by skin tone	More affected	Less affected
Accuracy in darker skin tone	More concerned	Less concerned

Abbreviation: CWST, consumer wearable sleep tracker.

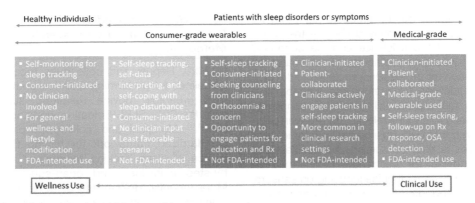

Fig. 1. Clinical scenarios in which wearables may be used.

scenarios, because clinicians were not consulted or involved in evaluating and treating sleep disturbances, which may have the unintended consequence of undiagnosed and, therefore, untreated sleep disorders. To our knowledge, the exact prevalence of this scenario has not been systemically explored, but it may be prevalent. Further investigation into this population may help us understand how best to encourage them to seek care.

Scenario #3: Patients with sleep disorders or symptoms using CWST for sleep-tracking with counseling from clinicians

Consumers using wearables under clinician guidance is a more desirable scenario, because it offers an excellent opportunity for clinicians to intervene in treating sleep disorders and actively engage patients in education. In this scenario, patients and clinicians can discuss the data and develop a plan for longitudinal monitoring, thus adding a new facet to their ongoing sleep evaluation. Notably, clinicians may encounter occasional patients with "orthosomnia," a condition where patients are excessively preoccupied, concerned with, or even anxious about improving/perfecting their CWST data.[111] These patients may be overly reliant on their CWSTs, and the obsession/compulsion may exacerbate their insomnia. Orthosomnia can pose unique challenges in CBT-I because their negative perception of sleep may be too strong to reframe through cognitive-behavioral modification.[107] The true prevalence of orthosomnia is unknown, and how clinicians should best approach and treat it remains largely uninvestigated.

Scenario #4: Patients with sleep disorders or symptoms using CWSTs for sleep tracking under the direction or supervision of clinicians

This situation is typically clinician-initiated or researcher-initiated with patient collaboration. It is most likely a situation where a researcher initiates a clinical study using CWST and recruits patients who collaborate. This scenario is likely to occur where clinicians/researchers are familiar with the strengths and limitations of specific CWSTs used in the study, as opposed to scenario #3, where clinicians may not be experienced with the particular CWST device worn by a patient. Another circumstance is when a clinician does not have access to medical-grade actigraphy and encourages patients with CWSTs to track their sleep with the intention of utilizing the CWST data to help manage sleep disorders. This scenario may become more common as the Philips Actiwatch series is discontinued after December 29, 2022.[112]

Scenario #5: Patients with sleep disorders or symptoms use a medical-grade wearable for sleep tracking under the direction of clinicians

The final scenario is also clinician- or researcher-initiated and patient-collaborated, using a medical-grade wearable. Clinicians may use a medical-grade wearable to screen or diagnose OSA, track physiological sleep data, or follow up on treatment response. There are several novel medical-grade wearables/software as medical devices (SaMDs) for OSA detection. Further discussion of these devices is beyond the scope of this article.

RECOMMENDATIONS FOR THE USE OF CONSUMER WEARABLE SLEEP TRACKER IN VARIOUS CLINICAL SCENARIOS

Given the increased sophistication of wearables, the line between consumer-grade and medical-grade devices is blurry at best. Presently, there are no professional society clinical practice guidelines on the appropriate use of either consumer-grade or medical-grade wearables. Position statements exist, but no practical algorithm for their use has been proposed despite the broad acceptance of the existence and the continued growth of wearable technology. This creates an obvious need for professional societies to develop clinical guidelines for using these technologies, balancing the exponential growth of technology with the need to provide relevant data-driven guidance. Given that performance analysis for individual devices is time-consuming, it is unlikely that specific advice for each new device will be created, but a general guide focusing on sensors, algorithms, and intended use. Our recommendations based on the above-mentioned clinical scenarios are summarized in **Table 6**.

CURRENT CONCERNS AND FUTURE CHALLENGES

In addition to the urgent need for clinical practice guidelines, there are looming concerns over inadequate CWST performance assessment, the lack of standardized performance research methodologies, growing digital health disparity, and effective regulation.

Manufacturers: Why is there a Lack of Performance Evaluation Studies?

The lack of high-quality performance research trials has always been a concern. There are innumerable CWSTs on the market, with varying claims about the capability of their products to improve sleep. Yet, most CWSTs are barely "validated" or have had their performance assessed objectively. In 2016, the AASM recognized the inadequacy of validation research and encouraged such research studies.[18] Despite the call for manufacturers to validate their devices, performance assessment research continues to lag behind patient needs (**Table 7**). Manufacturers are often reluctant to perform performance evaluation research because of concerns about (1) the prolongation of the product development phase; (2) post-market requirements such as compliance with the quality management system regulation; and (3) the costs of clinical trials and publications, which can be a serious concern in the early product development phase for small start-ups.[113,114] Currently, the validation process can negatively impact device manufacture, design upgrade, marketing, and sales. Recently, a comprehensive evaluation framework incorporating measurement verification, analytical validation, clinical validation, and clinical utility testing has emerged through the Digital Medicine Society (DiMe), aiming to foster the development of digital medicine technologies.[115,116]

Researchers: We Need Standardized Performance Evaluation Research Methodologies

In 2020, Depner and colleagues recommended guidelines for performing and interpreting results from wearable device research, summarized from the 2018 SLEEP meeting workshop discussion.[119] Menghini and colleagues proposed a standardized framework for testing the performance of sleep-tracking technology with step-by-step guidelines and open-source code.[120] More recently, deZambotti et al. recommended using standardized terminology and operationalizing standard performance outcome metrics for scientific publication to prevent data misinterpretation and facilitate comparison across technologies.[121] These endeavors are critical for laying a solid scientific foundation for future validation research, and these guidelines may become a widely accepted standard for assessing the performance of CWSTs.

Community: How Can We Improve Digital Health Disparities?

There are legitimate concerns that sleep technological acceleration can lead to unintentional consequences such as worsening health disparities in already under-resourced populations, such as racial or ethnic minorities.[122] It will be essential for researchers, public health practitioners, clinicians, innovators, and manufacturers to facilitate the development of CWSTs capable of accurately assessing sleep metrics and to validate their accuracy in community populations to eliminate health disparities. Acknowledging the racial bias in pulse oximetry is a positive step toward equity.[75–80] Still, it must be followed by technological improvements through manufacturers, adjustments of oversight policies by the regulating agencies, and fine-tuning of clinical algorithms in managing dark-skinned patients by clinicians and health care institutions to minimize these biases.[123] Dependence upon technology to participate in health care (telemedicine, clinician-initiated wearable technologies) can further disenfranchise those already negatively impacted by their inability to access technology.

Regulating Agencies: How Best to Oversee Consumer Wearable Sleep Trackers?

The FDA clearly states that registered devices are intended for general wellness and historically emphasizes safety over accuracy/efficacy. With the increasing blurriness between CWSTs and medical-grade devices and their growing

Table 6
Recommendations concerning wearable sleep tracker use based on various clinical scenarios

Scenario #1–5	Recommendations
Scenario #1: Healthy individuals; consumer-initiated; no clinician involvement; CWST	• Consumers should be mindful that there could be significant variations in performance concerning sleep–wake outcomes and sleep stage classification among CWST brands, models, and hardware/software generations. The performance of one CWST device cannot be extrapolated to another. • Consumers should understand that CWSTs tend to overestimate sleep and underestimate wake, and the accuracy in detecting wake may vary significantly. • Consumers should note that variability exists in CWSTs' sleep stage classification even in healthy young subjects. • Consumers should be aware that the pulse oximetry of most CWSTs has not been validated, and its accuracy remains a concern. • Consumers should know that PRV validity varies with CWST devices. The better-performing ones appear to provide valid measurements for healthy young adults. • Consumers should be aware that dark skin tones may affect the performance of CWSTs' pulse oximetry and PR.
Scenario #2: Patients with sleep disorders or symptoms; consumer-initiated; no clinician involvement; CWST	• Consumers should be aware that the sleep–wake outcomes and sleep stage classification of CWSTs may not be as accurate in patients with sleep disturbance. • Consumers with sleep disturbance should avoid over-relying on CWSTs for self-management of sleep disturbance. • Consumers with sleep disturbance should seek medical attention and receive appropriate management from clinicians.
Scenario #3: Patients with sleep disorders or symptoms; consumer-initiated; clinician-counseled; CWST	• Clinicians should only use the data derived from CWSTs of known good performance in the context of a comprehensive clinical sleep evaluation. • Clinicians should avoid relying on the physiological data derived from inadequately validated CWSTs for clinical decisions. • Clinicians should carefully discern the functionalities, mechanisms, signals, outputs, strengths, and limitations of CWST devices used by patients and provide proper counseling concerning CWST use. • Clinicians should discern that the evidence supporting the broader use of CWSTs in patients with sleep disorders remains scarce. • Clinicians should be aware that the newer models of some CWST brands have comparable or better specificity for wake and are probably at least equivalent to medical-grade actigraphy in healthy young adults. Early evidence also suggests that some CWST brands/models may be as good as medical-grade actigraphy in patients with chronic insomnia.

(continued on next page)

Table 6 (continued)	
Scenario #1–5	**Recommendations**
	• Clinicians should closely assess and follow up on patients with orthosomnia for further management.
Scenario #4: Patients with sleep disorders or symptoms; clinician- or researcher-initiated; patient-collaborated; CWST	• Clinicians/researchers should fully comprehend the performance, strengths, and limitations of the CWSTs employed in clinical research. • Clinicians/researchers should inform patients/research subjects about the FDA clearance status of the CWSTs and provide counseling and education concerning the proper use of the device.
Scenario #5: Patients with sleep disorders or symptoms; clinician- or researcher-initiated; patient-collaborated; medical-grade wearable device	• Clinicians should fully comprehend the performance, strengths, and limitations of the medical-grade wearables or SaMDs used in clinical settings or employed in research. • Clinicians should provide patients or research subjects with adequate counseling and education concerning the proper use of medical-grade wearable devices.

Abbreviations: CWST, consumer wearable sleep tracker; FDA, U.S. Food & Drug Administration; PR, pulse rate; SaMD, software as a medical device.

prevalence, the accuracy and usability of CWSTs will ultimately be a concern. Further discussion on how best to oversee CWSTs may become more relevant over time.[124]

Clinicians: Should Clinicians Utilize Consumer Wearable Sleep Tracker Sleep Data for Clinical Decision-Making?

Because clinicians are seeing more patients armed with CWST sleep data, it is rational to raise the question, "Should clinicians interpret and utilize CWST sleep data for clinical decision-making?" Clinicians may be unwilling to interpret CWST data for the following reasons: (1) feeling inadequately equipped to interpret them; (2) concerned about the inaccuracy of CWST data; (3) worried about the malpractice liability derived from using nonmedical-grade devices; or (4) unwilling to use CWST data because of the lack of reimbursement. These are legitimate concerns, but before some of these issues are resolved, clinicians must assess their own competency and comfort level to decide if they will interpret the CWST sleep data, which must always be performed in the context of a comprehensive clinical sleep evaluation. Clinicians will likely rely on professional societies to provide guidance and education.

Other concerns, such as CWST data quality assurance, data collection, data presentation, cybersecurity, privacy, and incorporation of CWST data into electronic medical records, will also need to be addressed.[107,117,118]

Future Trends

Though not yet on the market as of this writing, 2 new CWST rings have recently received much attention.[125–127] The Happy Ring includes electrodermal activity, PPG, accelerometry, and temperature sensors.[125] In a study by Grandner and colleagues, the Happy Ring achieved a specificity of 0.70 for wake using the "generalized" ML algorithm and 0.83 using the "personalized" algorithm in 36 healthy adults.[125] The personalized algorithm demonstrated improved accuracy over the generalized algorithm and other devices tested (Acti-Watch 2, Fitbit Charge 4, WHOOP 3.0, Oura ring V2), suggesting that adaptable, dynamic AI algorithms can enhance sleep detection accuracy. This adaptive AI-enabled approach is appealing and warrants further research. Also, the Evie ring, a new ring "designed for women" and capable of period and ovulation tracing, was reportedly seeking FDA pulse oximetry functionality clearance.[127] Furthermore, "earables", which can sense physiological signals including temperature, accelerometry, PPG, EEG, and ECG from external ear canal, are also promising and worth our attention.[128]

As CWST AI/ML/DL models improve, real-time sleep classification may eventually become

Table 7
Reasons why manufacturers are reluctant to perform validation research or seek FDA clearance

Reasons	Details
Delays	• The clinical validation process may take 2–3 y, which can lead to considerable delays in the development and marketing of products. • The FDA Class II submission and clearance process may take another 6–24 mo.
Product lifecycle	• Lifecycles of CWST are frequently short, often shorter than the clinical validation process, which makes validation irrelevant.
FDA oversight	• Under FDA oversight, a QMS must be established to track all the medical-grade devices sold. For post-market surveillance, manufacturers are required to report complaints, technical issues, performance concerns, adverse events, and safety issues, including injuries and deaths, to ensure quality and reduce the risk of devices.
Costs	• Clinical validation trials, FDA applications, and QMS all incur additional costs.
Disconnect	• Small start-up manufacturers may have difficulty connecting with researchers or institutes interested in conducting validation trials in the early phases of developing innovative products.

Abbreviations: CWST, consumer wearable sleep tracker; FDA, U.S. Food & Drug Administration; QMS, quality management system.

possible.[129,130] With the advancement of ML and the Internet of Things, interactive ML systems may open doors to the possibility of proactive interventions, such as changing the ambient lighting, sounds, or temperature in sleep, with consumers not consciously aware of the changes.[130]

Another growing area is using CWST to deliver sleep interventions to improve sleep outcomes.[131,132] Baron and colleagues, in a scoping review, suggested that opportunities exist to utilize CWSTs to improve existing cognitive behavior therapy and wellness programs.[131] A recent meta-analysis on the effect of wearable-delivered sleep interventions by Lai and colleagues indicated that wearable-delivered interventions may complement usual care to improve sleep outcomes.[132]

SUMMARY

Sleep technology continues to be innovative and alluring to clinicians and consumers. Their sophistication and accuracy continue to evolve and improve, allowing clinicians and researchers to obtain objective physiological sleep data. There is optimism that wearable technology will enhance the care of patients with sleep disorders, in addition to increasing awareness of the importance of sleep itself. These devices will likely become clinical devices once they demonstrate accuracy and reliability and can be utilized with confidence. We do not believe this threshold has yet been achieved, and at present, they should remain as wellness devices or be used in clinical research settings. As current technologies (such as the Actiwatch) are sunsetting, new ones will likely take their place, and we need to understand how best to deploy them clinically while being reassured that the data are accurate. If a clinician or researcher wishes to utilize wearables, the ones with the best performance data are preferred. As always, these data should be used with appropriate clinical context as part of a comprehensive sleep evaluation. As we attempt to navigate this ever-changing field, collaboration between clinicians, industry, researchers, and professional societies is essential.[133–135] Re-examining our current processes is also crucial, as technology simply evolves too quickly to adhere to dated assessments. Stakeholders will need to embrace innovation and develop new standards for performance assessment, address basic thresholds for acceptability, and consider practical aspects of incorporating these technologies into clinical care, such as privacy, data storage, reimbursement for review of these data, and legal aspects of patient-generated health data uploaded to the EMR. Collaboration and embracing change while prioritizing patient care are likely the best paths forward as we learn how to harness technology to better care for patients.

DISCLOSURE

Dr A. A. Chiang has received research grants from Belun Technology Company Limited and Night-Ware for conducting clinical research but has no financial conflicts of interest related to this topic. Dr S. Khosla is a consultant for BrainTrain2020 and has no financial conflicts of interest related to this topic.

REFERENCES

1. The Nobel Assembly at Karolinska Institutet. 2017 Nobel Prize in Physiology or Medicine. Available at: https://www.nobelprize.org/uploads/2018/06/press-39.pdf. Accessed December 18, 2022.
2. Castillo M. The 3 pillars of health. Am J Neuroradiol 2015;36:1–2.
3. Yetisen AK, Martinez-Hurtado JL, Ünal B, et al. Wearables in medicine. Adv Mater 2018;30(33):e1706910.
4. Dunn J, Runge R, Snyder M. Wearables and the medical revolution. Per Med 2018;15(5):429–48.
5. Perez-Pozuelo I, Zhai B, Palotti J, et al. The future of sleep health: a data-driven revolution in sleep science and medicine. NPJ Digit Med 2020;3:42.
6. Schutte-Rodin S, Deak MC, Khosla S, et al. Evaluating consumer and clinical sleep technologies: an American Academy of Sleep Medicine update. J Clin Sleep Med 2021;17(11):2275–82.
7. Vijayan V, Connolly JP, Condell J, et al. Review of wearable devices and data collection Considerations for Connected health. Sensors 2021;21(16):5589.
8. Kwon S, Kim H, Yeo WH. Recent advances in wearable sensors and portable electronics for sleep monitoring. iScience 2021;24(5):102461.
9. Rentz LE, Ulman HK, Galster SM. Deconstructing commercial wearable technology: Contributions toward accurate and free-living monitoring of sleep. Sensors 2021;21(15):5071.
10. Tobin SY, Williams PG, Baron KG, et al. Challenges and opportunities for Applying wearable technology to sleep. Sleep Med Clin 2021;16(4):607–18.
11. de Zambotti M, Cellini N, Menghini L, et al. Sensors Capabilities, performance, and Use of consumer sleep technology. Sleep Med Clin 2020;15(1):1–30.
12. Goldstein C. Current and future Roles of consumer sleep technologies in sleep medicine. Sleep Med Clin 2020;15(3):391–408.
13. Lujan MR, Perez-Pozuelo I, Grandner MA. Past, present, and future of Multisensory wearable technology to monitor sleep and circadian rhythms. Front Digit Health 2021;3:721919.
14. Topol EJ. High-performance medicine: the convergence of human and artificial intelligence. Nat Med 2019;25(1):44–56.
15. Fitbit. What's sleep score in the Fitbit app?. Available at: https://help.fitbit.com/articles/en_US/Help_article/2439.htm. Accessed December 18, 2022.
16. OURA. An Introduction to Your Sleep Score. Available at: https://support.ouraring.com/hc/en-us/articles/360025445574-An-Introduction-to-Your-Sleep-Score. Accessed December 18, 2022.
17. Garmin. What is the Sleep Score and Insights Feature on My Garmin Watch?. Available at: https://support.garmin.com/en-US/?faq=DWcdBazhr097VgqFufsTk8. Accessed December 18, 2022.
18. Khosla S, Deak MC, Gault D, et al. Consumer sleep technology: an American academy of sleep medicine position statement. J Clin Sleep Med 2018;14(5):877–80.
19. Penzel T, Glos M, Fietze I. New trends and new technologies in sleep medicine: expanding accessibility. Sleep Med Clin 2021;16(3):475–83.
20. Korkalainen H, Nikkonen S, Kainulainen S, et al. Self-applied home sleep recordings: the future of sleep medicine. Sleep Med Clin 2021;16(4):545–56.
21. McNicholas WT. Getting more from the sleep recording. Sleep Med Clin 2021;16(4):567–74.
22. Grandner MA, Lujan MR, Ghani SB. Sleep-tracking technology in scientific research: looking to the future. Sleep 2021;44(5):zsab071.
23. Chinoy ED, Cuellar JA, Huwa KE, et al. Performance of seven consumer sleep-tracking devices compared with polysomnography. Sleep 2021;44(5):zsaa291.
24. Chinoy ED, Cuellar JA, Jameson JT, et al. Performance of four commercial wearable sleep-tracking devices tested under unrestricted conditions at home in healthy young adults. Nat Sci Sleep 2022;14:493–516.
25. U.S. Food & Drug Administration. Apple ECG App De Novo Summary (DEN180044). Available at: https://www.accessdata.fda.gov/cdrh_docs/reviews/DEN180044.pdf. Accessed December 18, 2022.
26. U.S. Food & Drug Administration. Fitbit ECG App 510(k) (K200948). Available at: https://www.accessdata.fda.gov/cdrh_docs/pdf20/K200948.pdf. Accessed December 18, 2022.
27. U.S. Food & Drug Administration. General Wellness: Policy for Low Risk Devices. Available at: https://www.fda.gov/regulatory-information/search-fda-guidance-documents/general-wellness-policy-low-risk-devices. Accessed December 18, 2022.
28. Bandyopadhyay A, Goldstein C. Clinical applications of artificial intelligence in sleep medicine: a sleep clinician's perspective. Sleep Breath 2022;1–17.
29. Goldstein CA, Berry RB, Kent DT, et al. Artificial intelligence in sleep medicine: background and implications for clinicians. J Clin Sleep Med 2020;16(4):609–18.
30. Davies HJ, Williams I, Peters NS, et al. In-ear SpO2: a tool for wearable, Unobtrusive monitoring of Core blood oxygen saturation. Sensors 2020;20(17):4879.
31. Palotti J, Mall R, Aupetit M, et al. Benchmark on a large cohort for sleep-wake classification with

machine learning techniques. NPJ Digit Med 2019; 7(2):50.

32. Webster JB, Kripke DF, Messin S, et al. An activity-based sleep monitor system for ambulatory use. Sleep 1982;5(4):389–99.

33. Cole RJ, Kripke DF, Gruen W, et al. Automatic sleep/wake identification from wrist activity. Sleep 1992;15(5):461–9.

34. Sadeh A, Sharkey KM, Carskadon MA. Activity-based sleep-wake identification: an empirical test of methodological issues. Sleep 1994;17(3):201–7.

35. Esteva A, Robicquet A, Ramsundar B, et al. A guide to deep learning in healthcare. Nat Med 2019;25(1):24–9.

36. Korkalainen H, Aakko J, Duce B, et al. Deep learning enables sleep staging from photoplethysmogram for patients with suspected sleep apnea. Sleep 2020;43(11):zsaa098.

37. Altini M, Kinnunen H. The Promise of sleep: a multisensor approach for accurate sleep stage detection using the Oura ring. Sensors 2021;21(13):4302.

38. Strumpf Z, Gu W, Tsai C, et al. Belun Ring (Belun Sleep System BLS-100): deep learning-facilitated wearable enables obstructive sleep apnea detection, apnea severity categorization, and sleep stages classification in patients suspected of obstructive sleep apnea. Sleep Health, accepted for publication (in print).

39. Rupp TL, Balkin TJ. Comparison of Motionlogger Watch and Actiwatch actigraphs to polysomnography for sleep/wake estimation in healthy young adults. Behav Res Methods 2011;43(4):1152–60.

40. Zinkhan M, Berger K, Hense S, et al. Agreement of different methods for assessing sleep characteristics: a comparison of two actigraphs, wrist and hip placement, and self-report with polysomnography. Sleep Med 2014;15(9):1107–14.

41. Quante M, Kaplan ER, Cailler M, et al. Actigraphy-based sleep estimation in adolescents and adults: a comparison with polysomnography using two scoring algorithms. Nat Sci Sleep 2018;10:13–20.

42. Montgomery-Downs HE, Insana SP, Bond JA. Movement toward a novel activity monitoring device. Sleep Breath 2012;16(3):913–7.

43. de Zambotti M, Claudatos S, Inkelis S, et al. Evaluation of a consumer fitness-tracking device to assess sleep in adults. Chronobiol Int 2015;32(7):1024–8.

44. de Zambotti M, Baker FC, Willoughby AR, et al. Measures of sleep and cardiac functioning during sleep using a multi-sensory commercially-available wristband in adolescents. Physiol Behav 2016;158:143–9.

45. Beattie Z, Oyang Y, Statan A, et al. Estimation of sleep stages in a healthy adult population from optical plethysmography and accelerometer signals. Physiol Meas 2017;38(11):1968–79.

46. de Zambotti M, Goldstone A, Claudatos S, et al. A validation study of Fitbit Charge 2™ compared with polysomnography in adults. Chronobiol Int 2018;35(4):465–76.

47. Walch O, Huang Y, Forger D, et al. Sleep stage prediction with raw acceleration and photoplethysmography heart rate data derived from a consumer wearable device. Sleep 2019;42(12):zsz180.

48. Roberts DM, Schade MM, Mathew GM, et al. Detecting sleep using heart rate and motion data from multisensor consumer-grade wearables, relative to wrist actigraphy and polysomnography. Sleep 2020;43(7):zsaa045.

49. Miller DJ, Lastella M, Scanlan AT, et al. A validation study of the WHOOP strap against polysomnography to assess sleep. J Sports Sci 2020;38(22):2631–6.

50. de Zambotti M, Rosas L, Colrain IM, et al. The sleep of the ring: comparison of the ŌURA sleep tracker against polysomnography. Behav Sleep Med 2019;17(2):124–36.

51. Miller DJ, Sargent C, Roach GD. A validation of six wearable devices for estimating sleep, heart rate and heart rate variability in healthy adults. Sensors 2022;22(16):6317.

52. Kang SG, Kang JM, Ko KP, et al. Validity of a commercial wearable sleep tracker in adult insomnia disorder patients and good sleepers. J Psychosom Res 2017;97:38–44.

53. Kahawage P, Jumabhoy R, Hamill K, et al. Validity, potential clinical utility, and comparison of consumer and research-grade activity trackers in Insomnia Disorder I: in-lab validation against polysomnography. J Sleep Res 2020;29(1):e12931.

54. Dong X, Yang S, Guo Y, et al. Validation of Fitbit Charge 4 for assessing sleep in Chinese patients with chronic insomnia: a comparison against polysomnography and actigraphy. PLoS One 2022;17(10):e0275287.

55. Toon E, Davey MJ, Hollis SL, et al. Comparison of commercial wrist-based and smartphone accelerometers, actigraphy, and PSG in a clinical cohort of children and adolescents. J Clin Sleep Med 2016;12(3):343–50.

56. Gruwez A, Bruyneel AV, Bruyneel M. The validity of two commercially-available sleep trackers and actigraphy for assessment of sleep parameters in obstructive sleep apnea patients. PLoS One 2019;14(1):e0210569.

57. Moreno-Pino F, Porras-Segovia A, López-Esteban P, et al. Validation of Fitbit Charge 2 and Fitbit Alta HR against polysomnography for assessing sleep in adults with obstructive sleep apnea. J Clin Sleep Med 2019;15(11):1645–53.

58. Smith MT, McCrae CS, Cheung J, et al. Use of actigraphy for the evaluation of sleep disorders and circadian rhythm sleep-wake disorders: an American Academy of sleep medicine clinical practice guideline. J Clin Sleep Med 2018;14(7):1231–7.

59. Cook JD, Prairie ML, Plante DT. Ability of the Multisensory Jawbone UP3 to Quantify and classify sleep in patients with suspected central disorders of hypersomnolence: a comparison against polysomnography and actigraphy. J Clin Sleep Med 2018;14(5):841–8.

60. Lipnick MS, Feiner JR, Au P, et al. The accuracy of 6 Inexpensive pulse oximeters not cleared by the Food and Drug Administration: the possible global public health implications. Anesth Analg 2016; 123(2):338–45.

61. Kirszenblat R, Edouard P. Validation of the Withings ScanWatch as a wrist-worn reflective pulse oximeter: Prospective interventional clinical study. J Med Internet Res 2021;23(4):e27503.

62. Ryals S, Chiang A, Schutte-Rodin S, et al. Photoplethysmography (PPG)-new applications for an old technology: a sleep technology review. J Clin Sleep Med 2022. https://doi.org/10.5664/jcsm. 10300. Epub ahead of print.

63. Apple. How to use the Blood Oxygen app on Apple Watch. Available at: https://support.apple.com/en-us/HT211027. Accessed December 18, 2022.

64. Fitbit. How do I track blood oxygen saturation (SpO2) with my Fitbit device? Available at: https://help.fitbit.com/articles/en_US/Help_article/2459. htm. Accessed December 18, 2022.

65. U.S. Food & Drug Administration. Pulse oximeters - premarket notification submissions (510(k)s): guidance for industry and food and drug administration staff. US Food & Drug Administration. 2013. Mar. Available at: https://www.fda.gov/regulatory-information/search-fda-guidance-documents/pulse-oximeters-premarket-notification-submissions-510ks-guidance-industry-and-food-and-drug. Accessed December 18, 2022.

66. U.S. Food & Drug Administration. Withings Scan Monitor 510(k) (K201456). Available at: https://www.accessdata.fda.gov/cdrh_docs/pdf20/K201456.pdf. Accessed December 18, 2022.

67. Pipek L, Nascimento R, Acencio M, et al. Comparison of SpO_2 and heart rate values on Apple Watch and conventional commercial oximeters devices in patients with lung disease. Sci Rep 2021;11(1): 18901.

68. Spaccarotella C, Polimeni A, Mancuso C, et al. Assessment of non-Invasive measurements of oxygen saturation and heart rate with an Apple smartwatch: comparison with a standard pulse oximeter. J Clin Med 2022;11(6):1467.

69. Apple. Blood Oxygen app on Apple Watch. Available at: https://www.apple.com/healthcare/docs/site/Blood_Oxygen_app_on_Apple_Watch_October_2022.pdf. Accessed December 18, 2022.

70. Bodimetrics. Prevention circul+ Wellness Ring. Available at: https://bodimetrics.com/product/prevention-circul-wellness-ring/. Accessed December 18, 2022.

71. Rashid NH, Zaghi S, Scapuccin M, et al. The value of oxygen Desaturation Index for diagnosing obstructive sleep apnea: a systematic review. Laryngoscope 2021;131(2):440–7.

72. Zhao R, Xue J, Zhang X, et al. Comparison of ring pulse oximetry using reflective photoplethysmography and PSG in the detection of OSA in Chinese adults: a Pilot study. Nat Sci Sleep 2022;14:1427–36.

73. SLEEPON. Track your current body status. Available at: https://www.sleepon.us/app/. Accessed December 18, 2022.

74. SLEEPON. Understanding AHI – apnea-hypopnea index. Available at: https://www.sleepon.us/ahi/. Accessed December 18, 2022.

75. Sjoding MW, Dickson RP, Iwashyna TJ, et al. Racial bias in pulse oximetry measurement. N Engl J Med 2020;383(25):2477–8.

76. U.S. Food & Drug Administration. Pulse Oximeter Accuracy and Limitations: FDA Safety Communication. Available at: https://www.fda.gov/medical-devices/safety-communications/pulse-oximeter-accuracy-and-limitations-fda-safety-communication. Accessed December 18, 2022.

77. U.S. Food & Drug Administration. FDA Executive Summary: Review of Pulse Oximeters and Factors that can Impact their Accuracy. Available at: https://www.fda.gov/media/162709/download. Accessed December 18, 2022.

78. Cabanas AM, Fuentes-Guajardo M, Latorre K, et al. Skin pigmentation influence on pulse oximetry accuracy: a systematic review and Bibliometric analysis. Sensors 2022;22(9):3402.

79. Shi C, Goodall M, Dumville J, et al. The accuracy of pulse oximetry in measuring oxygen saturation by levels of skin pigmentation: a systematic review and meta-analysis. BMC Med 2022;20(1):267.

80. Poorzargar K, Pham C, Ariaratnam J, et al. Accuracy of pulse oximeters in measuring oxygen saturation in patients with poor peripheral perfusion: a systematic review. J Clin Monit Comput 2022; 36(4):961–73.

81. Shaffer F, Ginsberg JP. An Overview of heart rate variability metrics and Norms. Front Public Health 2017;5:258.

82. Almeida-Santos MA, Barreto-Filho JA, Oliveira JL, et al. Aging, heart rate variability and patterns of autonomic regulation of the heart. Arch Gerontol Geriatr 2016;63:1–8.

83. Stein PK, Pu Y. Heart rate variability, sleep and sleep disorders. Sleep Med Rev 2012;16(1):47–66.

84. Nunan D, Sandercock GRH, Brodie DA. A quantitative systematic review of normal values

for short-term heart rate variability in healthy adults. Pacing Clin Electrophysiol 2010;33:1407–17.

85. Li K, Rüdiger H, Ziemssen T. Spectral analysis of heart rate variability: time Window Matters. Front Neurol 2019;10:545.

86. Fang SC, Wu YL, Tsai PS. Heart rate variability and risk of all-cause death and cardiovascular events in patients with cardiovascular disease: a meta-analysis of cohort studies. Biol Res Nurs 2020; 22(1):45–56.

87. Tobaldini E, Nobili L, Strada S, et al. Heart rate variability in normal and pathological sleep. Front Physiol 2013;4:294.

88. Alvares GA, Quintana DS, Hickie IB, et al. Autonomic nervous system dysfunction in psychiatric disorders and the impact of psychotropic medications: a systematic review and meta-analysis. J Psychiatry Neurosci 2016;41(2):89–104.

89. Ucak S, Dissanayake HU, Sutherland K, et al. Heart rate variability and obstructive sleep apnea: current perspectives and novel technologies. J Sleep Res 2021;30(4):e13274.

90. Qin H, Steenbergen N, Glos M, et al. The different facets of heart rate variability in obstructive sleep apnea. Front Psychiatry 2021;12:642333.

91. Koch C, Wilhelm M, Salzmann S, et al. A meta-analysis of heart rate variability in major depression. Psychol Med 2019;49(12):1948–57.

92. Schneider M, Schwerdtfeger A. Autonomic dysfunction in posttraumatic stress disorder indexed by heart rate variability: a meta-analysis. Psychol Med 2020;50(12):1937–48.

93. Kang GE, Patriquin MA, Nguyen H, et al. Objective measurement of sleep, heart rate, heart rate variability, and physical activity in suicidality: a systematic review. J Affect Disord 2020;273:318–27.

94. Billman GE. The LF/HF ratio does not accurately measure cardiac sympatho-vagal balance. Front Physiol 2013;4:26.

95. Gil E, Orini M, Bailón R, et al. Photoplethysmography pulse rate variability as a surrogate measurement of heart rate variability during non-stationary conditions. Physiol Meas 2010;31(9):1271–90.

96. Mejía-Mejía E, May JM, Torres R, et al. Pulse rate variability in cardiovascular health: a review on its applications and relationship with heart rate variability. Physiol Meas 2020;41(7):07TR01.

97. Altini M. The Ultimate Guide to Heart Rate Variability (HRV): Part 1. Available at: https://medium.com/@altini_marco/the-ultimate-guide-to-heart-rate-variability hrv part-1-70a0a392fff4. Accessed December 18, 2022.

98. Pinheiro N, Couceiro R, Henriques J, et al. Can PPG be used for HRV analysis? Annu Int Conf IEEE Eng Med Biol Soc 2016;2016:2945–9.

99. OURA. An Introduction to Heart Rate Variability. Available at: https://support.ouraring.com/hc/en-us/articles/360025441974-An-Introduction-to-Heart-Rate-Variability. Accessed December 18, 2022.

100. BIPR. HRV Tracker app for Samsung Galaxy watches. Available at: https://bipr.fr/hrv-tracker-app-samsung-watch. Accessed December 18, 2022.

101. Altini M. Thoughts on Heart Rate Variability (HRV) measurement timing: morning or night? Available at: https://medium.com/@altini_marco/thoughts-on-heart-rate-variability-hrv-measurement-timing-morning-or-night-b92bd5495bc8. Accessed December 18, 2022.

102. Stone JD, Ulman HK, Tran K, et al. Assessing the accuracy of popular commercial technologies that measure resting heart rate and heart rate variability. Front Sports Act Living 2021;3:585870.

103. Lam E, Aratia S, Wang J, et al. Measuring heart rate variability in free-living conditions using consumer-grade photoplethysmography: validation study. JMIR Biomed Eng 2020;5(1):e17355.

104. Khandoker AH, Karmakar CK, Palaniswami M. Comparison of pulse rate variability with heart rate variability during obstructive sleep apnea. Med Eng Phys 2011;33(2):204–9.

105. Hoog Antink C, Mai Y, Peltokangas M, et al. Accuracy of heart rate variability estimated with reflective wrist-PPG in elderly vascular patients. Sci Rep 2021;11(1):8123.

106. Colvonen PJ, DeYoung PN, Bosompra NA, et al. Limiting racial disparities and bias for wearable devices in health science research. Sleep 2020; 43(10):zsaa159.

107. Nelson BW, Low CA, Jacobson N, et al. Guidelines for wrist-worn consumer wearable assessment of heart rate in biobehavioral research. NPJ Digit Med 2020;3:90.

108. Bent B, Goldstein BA, Kibbe WA, et al. Investigating sources of inaccuracy in wearable optical heart rate sensors. NPJ Digit Med 2020;3:18.

109. Berryhill S, Morton CJ, Dean A, et al. Effect of wearables on sleep in healthy individuals: a randomized crossover trial and validation study. J Clin Sleep Med 2020;16(5):775–83.

110. Khosla S, Wickwire EM. Consumer sleep technology: accuracy and impact on behavior among healthy individuals. J Clin Sleep Med 2020;16(5): 665–6.

111. Baron KG, Abbott S, Jao N, et al. Orthosomnia: are some patients taking the Quantified self too far? J Clin Sleep Med 2017;13(2):351–4.

112. Philips. Product discontinuation notice for Actiware, Actiwatch 2, Actiwatch PRO, and Actiwatch Plus. Available at: https://www.philips.com/c-dam/b2bhc/master/sites/actigraphy/product-eol-actigraphy-november-2023.pdf?_ga=2.268235854.1318015445.1672259325-386098475.1672259325. Accessed December 28, 2022.

113. Jiang N, Mück JE, Yetisen AK. The regulation of wearable medical devices. Trends Biotechnol 2020;38(2):129–33.

114. Chiang AA, Folz RJ. A subtle impediment to the progress of clinical sleep research. Sleep 2021; 44(10):zsab196.

115. Goldsack JC, Coravos A, Bakker JP, et al. Verification, analytical validation, and clinical validation (V3): the foundation of determining fit-for-purpose for Biometric Monitoring Technologies (BioMeTs). NPJ Digit Med 2020;3:55.

116. Digital Medicine Society (DiMe). Advancing Digital Medicine to Optimize Human Health. Available at: https://www.dimesociety.org/. Accessed December 18, 2022.

117. The Lancet Digital Health. Every breath you take, every move you make. Lancet Digit Health 2020; 2(12):e629.

118. Ash GI, Stults-Kolehmainen M, Busa MA, et al. Establishing a global standard for wearable devices in sport and exercise medicine: perspectives from Academic and industry stakeholders. Sports Med 2021;51(11):2237–50.

119. Depner CM, Cheng PC, Devine JK, et al. Wearable technologies for developing sleep and circadian biomarkers: a summary of workshop discussions. Sleep 2020;43(2):zsz254.

120. Menghini L, Cellini N, Goldstone A, et al. A standardized framework for testing the performance of sleep-tracking technology: step-by-step guidelines and open-source code. Sleep 2021; 44(2):zsaa170.

121. de Zambotti M, Menghini L, Grandner MA, et al. Rigorous performance evaluation (previously, "validation") for informed use of new technologies for sleep health measurement. Sleep Health 2022; 8(3):263–9.

122. Brewer LC, Fortuna KL, Jones C, et al. Back to the future: Achieving health equity through health Informatics and digital health. JMIR Mhealth Uhealth 2020;8(1):e14512.

123. Kupke A, Shachar C, Robertson C. Pulse oximeters and Violation of Federal Antidiscrimination Law. JAMA 2023. https://doi.org/10.1001/jama.2022.24976. Epub ahead of print.

124. Minen MT, Stieglitz EJ. Wearables for Neurologic conditions: Considerations for our patients and research limitations. Neurol Clin Pract 2021;11(4): e537–43.

125. Grandner MA, Bromberg Z, Hadley A, et al. Performance of a multisensor smart ring to evaluate sleep: in-lab and home-based evaluation of generalized and personalized algorithms. Sleep 2023 Jan 11;46(1):zsac152.

126. Happy Ring. Happy Ring feels what you feel. Available at: https://www.happyring.com. Accessed January 30, 2023.

127. Evie. Coming in 2023: The First Medical Grade Health Wearable Designed for Women. Available at: https://eviering.com. Accessed January 30, 2023.

128. Choi JY, Jeon S, Kim H, et al. Health-related Indicators measured using earable devices: systematic review. JMIR Mhealth Uhealth 2022;10(11):e36696.

129. van Berkel N, Skov MB, Kjeldskov J. Human-AI interaction. Interactions 2021;28(6):67e71.

130. Djanian S, Bruun A, Nielsen TD. Sleep classification using Consumer Sleep Technologies and AI: a review of the current landscape. Sleep Med 2022;100:390–403.

131. Glazer Baron K, Culnan E, Duffecy J, et al. How are consumer sleep technology data being used to deliver behavioral sleep medicine interventions? A systematic review. Behav Sleep Med 2022; 20(2):173–87.

132. Lai MYC, Mong MSA, Cheng LJ, et al. The effect of wearable-delivered sleep interventions on sleep outcomes among adults: a systematic review and meta-analysis of randomized controlled trials. Nurs Health Sci 2022. https://doi.org/10.1111/nhs.13011. Epub ahead of print.

133. Baumert M, Cowie MR, Redline S, et al. Sleep characterization with smart wearable devices: a call for standardization and consensus recommendations. Sleep 2022;45(12):zsac183.

134. Goldstein C, de Zambotti M. Into the wild the need for standardization and consensus recommendations to leverage consumer-facing sleep technologies. Sleep 2022;45(12):zsac233.

135. Devine JK, Schwartz LP, Hursh SR. Technical, regulatory, economic, and trust issues preventing successful integration of sensors into the Mainstream consumer wearables market. Sensors 2022;22(7): 2731.

Sleep Deficiency and Cardiometabolic Disease

Roo Killick, MBBS, FRACP, PhD[a], Lachlan Stranks, MBBS[a,b], Camilla M. Hoyos, MPH, PhD[a,c,*]

KEYWORDS

- Sleep restriction • Sleep deprivation • Cardiovascular disease • Cardiometabolic outcomes
- Metabolic health

KEY POINTS

- Short sleep duration has been associated with many negative cardiometabolic outcomes including mortality, coronary heart disease, and type 2 diabetes mellitus.
- Many underlying pathways have been proposed to link sleep deficiency and cardiometabolic dysfunction including oxidative stress, inflammation, endothelial dysfunction, and insulin resistance, which have been investigated in animal models and experimental human studies.
- Early evidence on whether sleep extension could reduce cardio-metabolic impacts of habitual sleep restriction is inconsistent and strategies on the implementation of such interventions still need to be developed.

INTRODUCTION

Sleep is a basic human need and lack of sleep disrupts many physiologic processes and health outcomes. Sleep loss has long been established to have widespread detrimental effects, with the earliest sleep deprivation experiments in rodents showing that the animals could not survive extreme durations of sleep deprivation, likely due to disturbances in cardiometabolic and immunologic control.[1] The National Sleep Foundation's most recent recommendations suggest that the ideal nightly duration of sleep for adults is between 7 and 9 h/night.[2] To date there have been numerous publications, suggesting that globally humans are sleeping less than previously, with a higher proportion of modern society curtailing their sleep due to various societal pressures.[3–5] Some have disputed this data due to discrepancies in how subjective sleep duration is assessed and the potential lack of correlation with objective sleep measurements.[6] Despite this, there is ample evidence, both experimental and at a population level, implicating sleep loss as a risk factor for negative cardiometabolic outcomes.[7,8] In this review we will summarize the main adverse cardiometabolic effects associated with sleep loss and discuss the mechanisms that are implicated within this relationship. For many of the outcomes, U-shaped relationships with sleep duration have been described; however, the associations with long sleep duration are outside the focus of this review. Furthermore, we will provide an overview of interventional studies examining the effect of short-term sleep extension on a variety of cardiometabolic outcomes.

CLINICAL OUTCOMES

Mortality, Cardiovascular Mortality, and Coronary Artery Disease

The association between sleep duration and overall mortality was first reported nearly 60 years ago[9] and has been confirmed in differing populations

This article originally appeared in *Clinics in Chest Medicine*, Volume 43 Issue 2, June 2022.

[a] Centre for Sleep and Chronobiology, Woolcock Institute of Medical Research, University of Sydney, Sydney, Australia; [b] The University of Adelaide, Faculty of Health and Medical Sciences, Adelaide, Australia; [c] The University of Sydney, Faculty of Science, School of Psychology and Brain and Mind Centre, Sydney, Australia
* Corresponding author. Woolcock Institute of Medical Research, PO Box M77, Missenden Road, New South Wales 2050, Australia.
E-mail address: camilla.hoyos@sydney.edu.au

Sleep Med Clin 18 (2023) 331–347
https://doi.org/10.1016/j.jsmc.2023.05.012
1556-407X/23/

since that time, including various recent meta-analyses and systematic reviews of the ever-growing literature in this area.[10–26] Many of these studies report a U-shaped relationship with sleep duration, and we will focus on the evidence that exists for short sleep duration for the purposes of this review. The associations with longer sleep duration could represent other pathophysiology, depending on the age and comorbidities of the population under investigation. Reports even suggest a gender difference in some of these relationships. Nonetheless most use 7 h/night as the reference point of so-called healthy sleep duration.

Coronary artery disease (CAD) is a significant cause of morbidity and mortality worldwide, and prevalence continues to rise.[27] Abnormal sleep duration has been identified as a risk factor for developing CAD in multiple epidemiologic studies,[28–30] and the U-shaped relationship once again is demonstrated in many, implicating both short and long sleep duration.[31–37] As an example of such data, a meta-analysis of 15 studies comprising 474,684 participants, demonstrated short sleep duration, defined as ≤5 to 6 h/night, was associated with an increased risk of developing or dying from CAD (relative risk (RR): 1.48, 95% confidence interval (CI): 1.22 to 1.80).[34] A prospective study of 60,586 Taiwanese adults similarly demonstrated that subjective sleep duration of less than 6 h/night significantly increased the risk of CAD in adults 40 years of age or older (hazards ratio (HR): 1.13, 95% CI: 1.04 to 1.23).[35] Interestingly, this study showed that individuals with subjective poor sleep quality were also at a higher risk of CAD compared with those who felt they had good quality sleep.[35] This finding is reflected in other work which demonstrated the risk of CAD was in fact highest in those with both short sleep duration and concurrent sleep disturbance (RR: 1.55, 95% CI: 1.33–1.81), with the risk being lower in people reporting only one of these anomalies.[36] It has been suggested that the higher incidence of type 2 diabetes mellitus found prospectively among short and long sleepers was one of, if not the primary, factor driving the paralleled increased risk of CAD in those with subjective short (<6 h/night) and long (>9 h/night) sleep duration in a cohort of 16,344 middle-aged men and women in the Malmö Diet Cancer Study followed for 14 to 16 years.[37] Diabetes is certainly an established risk factor for CAD; however, there are likely multiple pathophysiological mechanisms responsible for this positive association to which sleep restriction contributes. There is also an association between short sleep duration and risk of cardiac arrhythmias. In particular, the risk of atrial fibrillation has been shown to be higher in short sleepers in pooled observation studies.[38–41]

Hypertension

Sleep is associated with various physiologic alterations, including blood pressure control. Blood pressure is regulated through multiple mechanisms, including peripheral vascular resistance, cardiac contractility, and cardiac output. These mechanisms are largely regulated by the autonomic nervous system with 24h hemodynamic oscillations a result of fluctuating sympathetic and parasympathetic output.[42] During normal sleep, it is expected blood pressure will fall by at least 10% from daytime wake levels, a phenomenon referred to as the "nocturnal dip."[43,44] A pertinent finding in persistent short sleepers is the attenuation of this nocturnal blood pressure decline, and in turn increased daytime blood pressure.[43] As a result, there is increasing evidence, indicating that the blunting of the nocturnal blood pressure dip is associated with increased overall cardiovascular morbidity and mortality.[45] There are multiple physiologic processes likely responsible for this phenomenon, including increased sympathetic activity, increased catecholamine release,[46] an altered inflammatory response[44] and deranged circadian rhythm[47] which in turn could lead to increased daytime blood pressure.

Epidemiologic studies in well-established cohorts have demonstrated a relationship between short sleep duration and a higher prevalence of hypertension.[28,48–57] Some studies reported that the association between short sleep duration and hypertension was more pronounced in women and variable among different age groups. Results from the long-established, large Whitehall II cohort indicated only women were at higher risk of hypertension as a result of sleep deficiency, while no obvious pattern could be established in male subjects, when looking at cross-sectional analyses at the 12 to 14 year (phase 5) follow-up.[54] This finding was also reflected in a cohort of 3027 subjects in the Western New York Health Study showing women sleeping less than 6 h/night were at the highest risk of hypertension, with the effect being strongest in premenopausal women.[58] Interestingly, there may be a dose-dependent relationship between sleep duration and hypertension risk, with a shorter sleep duration more strongly associated with hypertension.[56] For instance, data from the Whitehall II study in their 5 year prospective analysis found those sleeping 6 h/night at 1.6 times (odds ratio (OR): 1.56 95% CI: 1.07–2.27), and those sleeping less than 5 h/night at nearly 2 times (OR: 1.94 95% CI: 1.08–3.50) greater risk of developing hypertension compared with those sleeping 7 h/night.[54]

A meta-analysis of 6 prospective and 17 cross-sectional studies confirmed the increased prevalence of hypertension (OR: 1.20, 95% CI: 1.09–1.32) with short sleep duration, especially in women and in subjects less than 65 years old.[52] As the collective data have grown in the past decade, further meta-analyses have been performed confirming that the relationship of short sleep duration holds with both prevalence and incidence of hypertension;[56,57,59] however, caution has been drawn to methodology when pooling results with regard to confounders and definitions of sleep duration cut-offs.[60]

Cerebrovascular Disease

Stroke is a significant cause of global morbidity and mortality. Numerous studies have investigated the relationship between short sleep duration and incidence of cerebrovascular disease.[28,61] For instance, results from a cohort of 266,848 Australian adults indicated a significantly increased risk of stroke in individuals sleeping less than 6 h/night (OR: 1.70, 95% CI: 1.50–1.92), compared with 7 h/night.[28] A recent meta-analysis of 20 studies assessing altered sleep duration and stroke risk demonstrated the lowest risk of stroke with a sleep duration of 6 to 7 h/night, and subsequent pooled relative risk of stroke of 1.05 (95% CI: 1.01–1.09) for every hour reduction of sleep beyond this.[62] This parallels a previous meta-analysis showing a J-shaped relationship between sleep duration and stroke or stroke mortality, with an increased relative risk of stroke events of 1.07 (95% CI: 1.02–1.12) for each hour reduction below 7 h/night. Interestingly, longer sleep duration was associated with a higher risk of stroke mortality, which may have different pathophysiologies in regard to those with significant illness and comorbidities.[63]

Obesity and Metabolic Syndrome

Sleep loss and its relationship with obesity have been long established, with ample epidemiologic data, suggesting that shorter sleepers have an increased risk of obesity across all age groups,[64–69] although there are likely differences between ethnicities.[70,71] A recent meta-analysis of prospective cohort studies found a reverse J-shape relationship with sleep duration; with a 9% increased risk of obesity seen for every hour reduction in sleep from 7 h/night.[72] Importantly with the growing obesity epidemic[73,74] and ever-increasing obesity rates,[75] there is particular

interest in children and adolescences,[76,77] hoping that sleep could be a modifiable risk factor in the development of obesity. A systematic review and meta-analysis of prospective longitudinal data in children from infancy to adolescence found the association held firm across all age groups.[78] There was also an inverse relationship between sleep duration and change in BMI over time.[78] More specifically another meta-analysis examined this exclusively in preschool children and again found a robust relationship between short sleep and the risk of developing obesity (RR: 1.54; 95% CI: 1.33–1.77) in 42,878 children across 13 studies). Furthermore in 4 out of 5 intervention studies analyzed, improved outcomes were seen with sleep extension.[79]

When exploring the components that would lead to the development of an increased cardiovascular risk profile, aside from obesity alone, sound epidemiologic data of over 45 studies have shown a relationship between short sleep and the incidence of the metabolic syndrome, a collection of cardiometabolic markers including blood pressure, waist circumference, lipid and glucose parameters.[80,81] For instance the Quebec Family Study, a cross-sectional study of 810 adults, found short sleepers (<6 h/night) had an increased risk of metabolic syndrome (OR: 1.76, 95% CI: 1.08–2.84) compared with 7–8 h/night after adjustment for various confounders.[82] This relationship was also confirmed in the large NHANES surveys.[83] Other data have reiterated this finding that men seem to be at higher risk than women in some domains,[84] whereas some have only found this relationship in extreme short sleepers (<4 h/night).[85] A study examined children and adolescents with similar results,[86] and data looking across all ages have suggested heterogeneity across differing age groups.[87] Bringing these examples and the wealth of similar literature together, a recent meta-analysis of both 36 cross-sectional and 9 longitudinal studies (n = 164,799 subjects and 430,895 controls) confirmed the relationship, in both prevalence (OR: 1.11, 95% CI: 1.05–1.18) and incidence (RR: 1.16, 95% CI: 1.05–1.23) of metabolic syndrome.[88] This review followed many similar meta-analyses,[89–92] which reflects the scientific interest in this subject, reinforcing the significant risk of cardiometabolic disease and the global importance to find ways to reduce its mortality and morbidity.

Diabetes Mellitus and Insulin Resistance

Similar data exist when exploring the incidence of type 2 diabetes mellitus and short sleep duration. Once again, the field is abloom with meta-analyses in the past decade illustrating this relationship, examining cross-sectional and prospective datasets across multiple population groups,[93–97] and furthermore looking specifically at glycemic control.[98] Type 2 diabetes has had much of the attention, but there is also a relationship between short sleep duration and glycemic control in type 1 diabetes,[99,100] with a meta-analysis describing 22 studies showing that children with type 1 diabetes had subjective shorter sleep than controls without diabetes.[100] In adults, although subjective sleep duration was not different between subjects and controls, there was better glycemic control (as determined by lower HbA1C levels) in those who slept >6 h/night compared with <6 h/night. There was also a higher incidence of poor sleep quality reported in those with higher HbA1C levels and a higher incidence of OSA.[100] Furthermore, the relationship with sleep duration has also been demonstrated in meta-analyses looking at gestational diabetes.[101,102]

PATHWAYS AND EXPERIMENTAL DATA

In this section, some of the proposed mechanistic pathways that may contribute toward the associations between short sleep duration and poor cardiometabolic outcomes will be explored. These include endothelial dysfunction, oxidative stress, and inflammatory pathways. Much of this cellular evidence has been performed in animal models; however, experimental trials in humans under tightly controlled sleep conditions have provided specific associations between sleep and metabolic outcomes and these will also be reviewed.

Endothelial Dysfunction

There is increasing evidence linking sleep deprivation with endothelial dysfunction, a known risk factor for cardiovascular disease.[103] Impairment of endothelium-dependent vasodilation is the hallmark of endothelial dysfunction, and while its pathogenesis in sleep restriction is likely multifactorial, sympathetic activation and reduced bioavailability of nitric oxide are likely critical. Animal studies have demonstrated that persistent sleep fragmentation in mice results in endothelial dysfunction and structural vascular change.[104] Doppler flow through the dorsal tail vein of mice was observed to alter after 8 to 9 weeks of persistent sleep disturbance, with reduction in peak blood flow from baseline, and increased duration of postocclusive hyperemic changes. Histologically, significant aortic structural changes were also found with elastic fiber disruption and disorganization, and immune cell infiltration, without significant change in wall thickness.[104] Experimental studies of sleep restriction in humans have also demonstrated impairment in markers of endothelial function mostly measured by flow-mediated brachial artery vasodilation (FMD).[105–107]

Oxidative Stress

Oxidative stress occurs when pro-oxidative pathways saturate antioxidant systems, resulting in an increased production of damaging reactive oxygen species (ROS). When this imbalance between these 2 systems generates an excess of these free radicals, a cascade of pro-inflammatory pathways can be initiated, leading to cellular damage and, over time, inflammation and subsequently, disease states can ensue. One proposed function of sleep is to remove ROS from the brain and other organs, and thus protect against oxidative injury.[108] Hence, sleep restriction may allow the accumulation of ROS and predispose to cellular injury.[109]

Experimental studies in this area are mostly described in animal models, as they are difficult to perform in humans. A meta-analysis of 44 animal studies supports that experimental sleep restriction in rodents promotes oxidative stress.[110] Furthermore, data demonstrate that sleep deprivation results in intestinal ROS accumulation in both flies and mice and may result in early mortality. It was suggested that this could be a consequence of alterations in the gut microbiota and modulation of gut immunity, disorders of which are also becoming increasingly implicated in human disease states.[111]

Studies in humans have similarly explored whether sleep deprivation contributes to the production of markers of oxidative stress, with some of the literature in this area performed in the context of intense physical activity. A study of 23 male students showed that after 36h of survival training, levels of lipid hydroperoxides and creatine kinase were elevated, but subsequently recovered after a single 12h period (only incorporating 7.5 h available sleep time).[112] In contrast, in a subsequent study of 15 soldiers who completed 48h of military survival training incorporating sleep deprivation (total sleep deprivation within first 24h and 3h sleep maximum in second 24h) showed reduced levels of glutathione peroxidase activity (that is reduced antioxidant activity), but no changes in the activity of other biochemical markers of oxidative stress, including lipid hydroperoxides, creatine kinase, and superoxide dismutase.[113]

Arrhythmogenicity

Experimental studies have also attempted to investigate the relationship between sleep duration, cardiac function, and arrhythmias. In a study of 27 healthy young adults subjected to acute sleep deprivation, echocardiographic assessment demonstrated reduced left atrial early diastolic strain rate,[114] suggesting that chronic sleep deprivation may produce more permanent alterations in the left atrium, and so predispose to atrial fibrillation and other atrial tachyarrhythmias.[114] Similarly, one night of sleep deprivation in healthy young individuals was associated with the prolongation of the QT interval, a phenomenon associated with higher risk of sudden cardiac death and ventricular tachyarrhythmias.[115] Intervention studies in humans have looked at cardiac autonomic changes with sleep deprivation. Sixty subjects had continuous ambulatory electrocardiogram monitoring and underwent 24h total sleep deprivation.[116] Significantly lower vagal activity and elevated sympathetic activity were found using heart rate variability, which improved after treatment with metoprolol. Furthermore, a randomized, placebo-controlled study of 72 healthy, young participants examined the effect of a statin on heart rate variability (as a marker of cardiac autonomic control) using a well-controlled in-laboratory study of 48h of total sleep deprivation. The addition of a statin led to a significant decrease in premature atrial and ventricular complexes, hence the authors promoted the concept of possible preventative cardiovascular treatment of those individuals at risk of sleep deprivation.[117]

Metabolomics and Transcriptomics

At a molecular level, there is much interest in the interaction between oxidative stress, metabolic markers, clock genes, and subsequent dysregulation by sleep loss. To attempt to understand the molecular mechanisms between sleep loss and metabolic dysregulation, studies have conducted metabolite profiling in the context of sleep loss to elucidate any markers of interest. In the first study which examined 12 healthy young male subjects undergoing 24h of total sleep deprivation, 27 out of a total of 171 metabolites had increased levels in the context of sleep loss, with 78 (out of 109) showing decreased amplitude in their circadian rhythmicity.[118] In a study investigating sleep restriction as opposed to total sleep deprivation, 2 metabolites (oxalic acid and diacylglycerol 36:3) were reduced following sleep restriction and restored following recovery in both rats and humans, suggesting a potential use as biomarkers of oxidative stress during sleep loss. Furthermore, higher levels of phospholipids were seen in both rodents and humans in this study, providing evidence of an oxidative environment.[119]

A landmark paper provided a comprehensive analysis of the effect of sleep loss on the human transcriptome.[120] Blood RNA samples were examined from 26 participants before and after a week of partial sleep deprivation (5.7 h/night (experimental arm) v 8.5 h/night (control arm)). This showed that an impressive 711 genes were up- or down-regulated by sleep loss, and these genes were associated with circadian rhythm, sleep homeostasis, metabolism, and oxidative stress, providing evidence that there are close relationships between all these circadian and physiologic processes.[120]

Inflammatory pathways

Various inflammatory pathways are upregulated in response to sleep deprivation, with effects on proinflammatory gene expression and increased levels of circulating inflammatory mediators.[121] Atherosclerosis is acknowledged as an inflammatory condition driven by circulating lipids and leukocytes and is a critical pathologic mechanism behind myocardial infarction and cerebrovascular disease through the formation of unstable arterial plaques.[122] Leukocytosis is a recognized predictor of cardiovascular events through white blood cells' role in the formation of these arterial lesions.[123]

A study demonstrated the relationship between sleep restriction and accelerated atherosclerosis in a population of mice predisposed to atherosclerotic disease. Compared with control mice, sleep-deprived mice were found to have more severe and extensive atherosclerotic disease despite no differences in body weight, glucose tolerance, or plasma cholesterol, but with higher levels of circulating leukocytes, particularly atherosclerosis-forming monocytes. Interestingly, reduced levels of hypocretin, the wakefulness-promoting protein, were found. This neuropeptide normally inhibits and regulates the release of colony-stimulating factor-1 (CSF-1) from neutrophil precursors, thus its deficiency results in increased production of CSF-1, and subsequently leukocytosis from the bone marrow.[124] Genetically altered mice who were unable to produce hypocretin similarly demonstrated more severe atherosclerosis, with reversal of this phenomenon following hypocretin administration, thus it was postulated sleep restriction results in signaling to the bone marrow to increase white blood cell production, ultimately damaging blood vessels.[124]

Increasing carotid intima-media thickness (CIMT) is a marker for subclinical coronary atherosclerosis and predictor of cardiac and cerebrovascular events in humans, given it reflects arterial inflammation.[125] In an observational cohort of

617 middle-aged adults, shorter sleep duration, measured objectively by actigraphy, was associated with increased CIMT in men but not women.[125] A subsequent systematic review explored the association between subjectively and objectively measured sleep duration and subclinical measures of cardiovascular disease including coronary artery calcium, carotid intima-media thickness, arterial stiffness, and endothelial dysfunction.[126] The association between short sleep duration (both subjective and objective) with CIMT had been consistently reported; however, the association with other surrogate markers was variable. The authors concluded, however, that despite the mixed results between the surrogate markers, there is a relationship between sleep duration at both extremes and subclinical cardiovascular burden.[126]

Small experimental human studies have investigated the relationship between partial sleep deprivation and circulating markers of inflammation and have demonstrated increased upstream proinflammatory activity and signaling in sleep restriction.[121,127] Conversely, a recent meta-analysis did not demonstrate an association between short sleep duration (<7 h/night) and elevated downstream systemic inflammatory markers, including C-reactive protein (CRP) and interleukin-6 (IL-6), suggesting that other mechanisms may also be contributing, or longer-term sleep restriction is required to demonstrate an elevation in measurable levels of proinflammatory markers.[128]

Insulin resistance, energy expenditure, weight gain

Several mechanisms to explain the relationship between short sleep duration, obesity and diabetes have been proposed, including higher calorific intake due to increased time awake, differences in energy expenditure, differences in eating behaviors, or changes in metabolic markers leading to cardiometabolic derangement. To investigate these mechanisms individually requires experimental studies with a high level of control of confounders. This ultimately translates to small, expensive to run, mainly in-laboratory studies, with strict sleep and environmental conditions.

A landmark paper was the first to establish that experimental sleep restriction led to reduced glucose tolerance in 11 healthy men sleep restricted to 4 h/night over 6 nights compared with post 6 nights of recovery sleep of 12 h/night.[129] As then many have replicated these findings, using different protocols and durations of sleep restriction,[130–137] which we and others have previously reviewed.[66,138,139] Data from our group explored whether this effect was also seen

in those individuals who catch-up on sleep at weekends and self-restrict during the working week, which is a prevalent sleep pattern in modern society.[140] Indeed, a similar reduction in insulin sensitivity was seen after extended partial sleep restriction compared with a weekend of sleep extension.[140]

Energy expenditure has also been examined under certain conditions to see whether that would explain the association of short sleep with weight gain. One such study under strict conditions in 16 individuals showed that after 5 days of sleep restriction, although energy expenditure increased by 5%, energy intake increased in excess of this leading to a positive energy balance and weight gain, particularly in women.[141] A study which measured energy expenditure by whole room calorimetry concurred with these findings.[142] Other data found similar changes in energy intake, but no change in energy expenditure.[143] A larger study also showed that food intake increased and weight was gained after 5 nights of sleep restriction, with higher intake of fat during the extra night time hours awake.[144] As those data were published, more studies followed, providing data for 2 meta-analyses of up to 18 studies.[145,146] One of these reports confirmed that increased energy intake occurs following sleep restriction without finding a change in energy expenditure, leading to an overall positive energy balance,[146] whereas the other meta-analysis showed that both energy expenditure and energy intake increased and the net result was less clear.[145] This ambiguity is not altogether surprising, as there are various ways to measure many of the variables in these experiments, alongside the small numbers of participants in the studies, encompassing both genders which may also cause differences in appetite regulation.[147] Indeed, there are also likely individual differences in energy metabolism.[148] However, taken overall these findings may postulate that there are likely both physiologic and behavioral components which lead to the increased food intake under conditions of sleep restriction,[149,150] and mechanistically these will lead to weight gain over time.

SLEEP EXTENSION STUDIES

With the mounting evidence of the association between short sleep duration and an increased risk of cardiometabolic health outcomes, interventions to reverse these complications need to be developed. Studies have investigated the effect of sleep extension; however, to date these have been of small sample size, with varying study designs and outcomes **Table 1**.[151–155]

Table 1
Sleep extension studies

	N; Age: Description	Design	Intervention	Outcomes	Findings (Reporting TST and Cardiometabolic Outcomes Only)
Al Khatib, 2018[1]	42; 18–64y; short sleep duration (5 to <7h-actigraphy)	RCT parallel, free-living	Sleep extension: 4 wk, behavioral consultation session on sleep hygiene Control: 4 wk, maintained habitual short sleep	Primary: feasibility and sugar intake Secondary: energy expenditure (RMR), body composition (bioelectric impedance), physical activity, anthropometry, lipids, appetite hormones, and HRV	Sleep extension ↑ TST by 21 mins (mean of 7 nights actigraphy). Sleep extension reduced intake of free sugars compared with control (Cohen's d = 0.79). No significant differences between groups in any secondary outcomes.
Baron, 2019[2]	16; 30–65y; pre/stage 1 hypertension (blood pressure ≥ 120–159/80–99 mm Hg on 24h ABPM) and <7h sleep duration (actigraphy)	RCT parallel (2:1 ratio), free-living	Sleep extension (n = 11): 6 wk, technology-assisted intervention Control (n = 5): 6 wk, self-management	Feasibility, 24h blood pressure	90% completion rate of coaching sessions, with enjoyment rated as 4 or 5/5. Sleep extension ↑ TST by 0.57 h and control ↑ by 0.08 h (actigraphy). Overall 24h SBP and DBP had greater reductions with sleep extension compared with the control. No other differences in other ABPM outcomes. No changes in BMI or office blood pressure measures.

(continued on next page)

Table 1
(continued)

	N; Age; Description	Design	Intervention	Outcomes	Findings (Reporting TST and Cardiometabolic Outcomes Only)
Haack, 2013[3]	22; 25–65y; h pre/stage 1 hypertension (120–159/80–99 mm Hg) and sleep duration <7h or sleep duration >1h shorter than self-estimated sleep need (sleep diaries and actigraphy)	RCT parallel, free-living	Sleep extension: 6 wk, bedtimes 30 min earlier and 30 min later than usual lights out/lights on times Control: 6 wk, continue habitual bedtimes	Primary: Beat to beat BP over 24h (digital photoplethysmography) Secondary: Nutrient intake (food records), weight, body fat (bioelectric impedance)[1], BMI, IL-6, hs-CRP, urinary creatinine, and norepinephrine	Sleep extension ↑ TST by 31 mins cf to control (actigraphy), SBP/DBP reduction of 14/8 mm Hg. No change in BMI, body fat, calorific intake, WBC, IL-6, CRP, norepinephrine.
Hartescu, 2021[4]	18; 25–55y; BMI >25 kg/m², sleep duration ≤6.5 h (actigraphy)	RCT parallel, free-living	Sleep extension: 6 wk, n = 10, program based on cognitive-behavioral principles Control: 6 wk, n = 8	Primary: TST (actigraphy) Secondary: Fasting plasma insulin, insulin resistance (HOMA-IR), blood pressure, appetite-related hormones from a mixed-meal tolerance test, continuous glucose levels.	Sleep extension ↑ TST by 72 min cf to controls (actigraphy). Sleep extension improved SBP, DBP, fasting insulin, HOMA-IR. No changes seen in weight, mean continuous glucose levels, fasting glucose, glucose AUC, fasting ghrelin, ghrelin AUC, fasting leptin levels.
Leproult, 2015[5]	16; 20–50y; BMI <30 kg/m². sleep duration <7h weekdays (sleep diaries and actigraphy)	Within-participant (before and after intervention), free-living	2 wk of habitual TIB, then 6 wk sleep extension (increasing TIB by 1 h/ night with sleep hygiene information and individual schedules)	TST (PSG, actigraphy), weight, fasting glucose, fasting insulin, insulin resistance (insulin-to-glucose ratio and HOMA), insulin sensitivity (QUICKI).	Sleep extension ↑ TST by 49 min (PSG, actigraphy). No changes in weight, glucose, or insulin levels. Correlations (n = 15) found associations between change in sleep time (actigraphy) and fasting glucose (r = +0.65, P = .017) insulin (r = −0.57, P = .053), insulin-to-glucose ratio (r = −0.66, P = .019) and QUICKI (r = 0.57, P = .053).

	Participants	Design	Intervention	Outcomes	Results
Moreno-Frais, 2020[6]	52; 14–18y; BMI <30 kg/m²	RCT Parallel, free-living	All calorie restricted by 500 cal/d. Sleep extension: 4 wk, (n = 25), personalised sleep plan to increase TST by 1h. Control: 4 wk (n = 27)	TST (sleep diaries), weight, glucose, insulin, insulin resistance (HOMA), lipid profile, leptin.	Weight decreased in both groups with diet. Sleep extension: ↑TST by 66 min (+36 min cf to controls), ↓weight, ↓waist circumference, ↓insulin, ↓IL6 cf to controls. No change in leptin, HOMA-IR.
Reutrakal, 2020[7] (sub-analysis of Son-ngern)	See later in discussion	See later in discussion	See later in discussion	Gut microbiota	No changes associated with sleep extension.
Reynold, 2014[8]	14; 18–55y, sleep duration 6–9h (self-report)	RCT, parallel, free-living	Sleep extension: 1 wk, n = 8, fixed sleep schedule whereby TIB was 3 h/night longer than the median baseline TIB (actigraphy) Control: 1 wk, n = 6	Physical activity (pedometer), blood pressure, heart rate, IL-6, TNF-α, CRP, and adiponectin	Sleep extension ↑TIB 127 min, TST 120 min Controls ↓TIB 27 min, TST 16 min (actigraphy). No changes between groups in blood pressure, heart rate, blood, except IL-6 which increased with extension but not control. Physical activity increased in both groups.
So-ngern, 2019[9]	21; 20–55y, self-reported ≤6h weekdays; nondiabetic (screening OGTT)	Cross-over (alternate order), free-living	Sleep extension: 2 wk, modifying bedtime earlier with individualized information. Control: 2 wk	Primary: OGTT -glucose metabolism (FBG, AUC glucose, insulin resistance [HOMA-IR], early insulin secretion [insulinogenic index], insulin sensitivity [Matsuda index], β-cell function [disposition index]) Secondary outcomes: self-reported sleep assessment (ESS, PSQI), dietary intake, weight.	Sleep extension ↑TST 36 mins (actigraphy). No changes in any outcomes with sleep extension cf to control. No order effect seen for glucose outcomes or the change in sleep duration itself. In those who slept >6h (n = 8) significant improvements seen in insulin resistance, early insulin secretion, and β-cell function.

(continued on next page)

Table 1
(continued)

	N; Age; Description	Design	Intervention	Outcomes	Findings (Reporting TST and Cardiometabolic Outcomes Only)
Stock, 2020[10]	53; 18–23y, undergraduate students; sleep duration 6–8h (actigraphy)	Within-participant (before and after intervention), free-living	Sleep extension: 1 wk, ↑TIB by 1h Control: 1 wk	Blood pressure, heart rate.	Sleep extension ↑TST 43 mins (actigraphy). Systolic BP ↓ sitting (−7.0 mm Hg ± 3.0, $P < .5$) and standing (−8.8 ± 2.7, $P < .1$). No changes in diastolic BP or heart rate.
Tasali, 2014[11]	10; 21–40y, BMI 25–<30 kg/m², sleep duration <6.5 h (self-report)	Within-participant (before and after intervention), free-living	Baseline: 1 wk, habitual TIB, followed by Sleep extension: 2 wk, ↑ TIB to 8.5 h, individualized behavioral counseling on sleep hygiene, with individual recommendations.	Appetite (visual analog scale), food desire (self-reported scales for different food items). Sleepiness (ESS),	Sleep extension ↑ TST 1.6 h (actigraphy). Sleep extension ↓overall appetite by 14% and desire for sweet/salty foods by 62%. Desire for fruit, vegetables, and protein-rich nutrients were not changed. Sleep extension ↓sleepiness, ↑vigor ratings.

[1] ABPM: ambulatory blood pressure monitoring; AUC: area under the curve; BMI: body mass index; CRP: C-reactive protein; DBP: diastolic blood pressure; ESS: Epworth sleep scale; FBG: fasting blood glucose; h: hours; HOMA-IR: HOMA-IR (Homeostatic Model Assessment for Insulin Resistance); HRV: heart rate variability; IL-6: Interleukin 6; min: minute; mmHg: millimetre of mercury; OGTT: oral glucose tolerance test; PSG: polysomnography; PSQI: Pittsburgh sleep quality index; QUICKI: quantitative insulin sensitivity check index; RCT: randomised controlled trial; RMR: resting metabolic rate; SBP: systolic blood pressure; TIB: time in bed; TNF: tumour necrosis factor; TST: total sleep time; WBC: white blood cells; wk: week; y: years.

Depending on the methodology chosen, some earlier experimental studies could be considered sleep extension studies relative to prior sleep deprivation; however, in general in many of those studies the individuals were often recruited as "normal" sleepers. This provides useful information with regards to putative target outcomes but may not physiologically be the same as trying to extend the sleep in habitual short sleepers, a population whom, as we have discussed in this review, are already at higher risk of cardiometabolic comorbidities.

Therefore, more recent studies (see **Table 1**) have specifically recruited the target population of habitual short sleepers and examined the feasibility of promoting and achieving longer sleep times. These have included advising earlier bedtimes or later wake-up times, sleep hygiene education, individualized sleep schedules, or even CBT techniques.[156–166] Many of the studies are still small in numbers and to our knowledge, there have not yet been large scale field studies to determine whether sleep extension interventions are practical and achievable at a population level. Using everyday technology such as activity monitors, and other wearables, now so widely available at relatively low cost, may be a way to provide this on a broader platform and in home environments.[164] While the results of these trials demonstrate variable and at times conflicting results, the intervention period in most of these studies has tended to be of relatively short duration (days to weeks). It is encouraging that all have used objective sleep measurements to document the increase in sleep duration, rather than self-report. Furthermore, these studies have all been in free-living conditions, not in sleep laboratories. Despite this meaning some confounders will be less controlled for, these studies are now very valuable to see if meaningful outcomes can be achieved in real-life settings. Thus, it remains to be seen whether longer-term sleep extension in larger sample sizes can reverse the negative effects of sleep restriction and improve cardiometabolic health outcomes.

SUMMARY

The cardiometabolic effects of short sleep duration are widely acknowledged and have been thoroughly examined in the literature over the past decade with ample meta-analyses of the available data encompassing many fields. The next step is how to broaden sleep extension studies to larger sample sizes so that any consistent benefits derived from lengthening sleep can help deliver sleep health recommendations at a population level.

CLINICS CARE POINTS

Sleep deprivation is associated with negative cardiometabolic outcomes.

- Asking about sleep duration should be incorporated into clinical discussions by health professions with individuals.
- Educating individuals about the importance of sleep as an overall general health measure is a clinical priority.

DISCLOSURES

The authors have no disclosure to declare.

FUNDING

Dr C. Hoyos is supported by a National Heart Foundation Future Leader Fellowship.

REFERENCES

1. Everson CA, Bergmann BM, Rechtschaffen A. Sleep deprivation in the rat: III. Total sleep deprivation. Sleep 1989;12(1):13–21.
2. Hirshkowitz M, Whiton K, Albert SM, et al. National Sleep Foundation's sleep time duration recommendations: methodology and results summary. Sleep Health 2015;1(1):40–3.
3. Jean-Louis G, Williams NJ, Sarpong D, et al. Associations between inadequate sleep and obesity in the US adult population: analysis of the national health interview survey (1977-2009). BMC Public Health 2014;14:290.
4. Basner M, Fomberstein KM, Razavi FM, et al. American time use survey: sleep time and its relationship to waking activities. Sleep 2007;30(9):1085–95.
5. Statistics NCfH. Quick-Stats: percentage of adults who reported an average of <6 hrs sleep per 24-hr period, by sex and age group- United States, 1985 and 2004. MMWR Morb Mort Wkly Rep 2005;54:933.
6. Bin YS, Marshall NS, Glozier N. Sleeping at the limits: the changing prevalence of short and long sleep durations in 10 countries. Am J Epidemiol 2013;177(8):826–33.
7. Cappuccio FP, Miller MA. Sleep and cardiometabolic disease. Curr Cardiol Rep 2017;19(11):110.
8. St-Onge MP, Grandner MA, Brown D, et al. Sleep duration and quality: impact on lifestyle behaviors and cardiometabolic health: a scientific statement

from the american heart association. Circulation 2016;134(18):e367–86.

9. Hammond EC. Some preliminary findings on physical complaints from a prospective study of 1,064,004 men and women. Am J Public Health Nations Health 1964;54:11–23.

10. Gangwisch JE, Heymsfield SB, Boden-Albala B, et al. Sleep duration associated with mortality in elderly, but not middle-aged, adults in a large US sample. Sleep 2008;31(8):1087–96.

11. Patel SR, Ayas NT, Malhotra MR, et al. A prospective study of sleep duration and mortality risk in women. Sleep 2004;27(3):440–4.

12. Grandner MA, Hale L, Moore M, et al. Mortality associated with short sleep duration: the evidence, the possible mechanisms, and the future. Sleep Med Rev 2010;14(3):191–203.

13. Wingard DL, Berkman LF. Mortality risk associated with sleeping patterns among adults. Sleep 1983; 6(2):102–7.

14. Tamakoshi A, Ohno Y. Self-reported sleep duration as a predictor of all-cause mortality: results from the JACC study, Japan. Sleep 2004;27(1):51–4.

15. Shankar A, Koh WP, Yuan JM, et al. Sleep duration and coronary heart disease mortality among Chinese adults in Singapore: a population-based cohort study. Am J Epidemiol 2008;168(12): 1367–73.

16. Kripke DF, Garfinkel L, Wingard DL, et al. Mortality associated with sleep duration and insomnia. Arch Gen Psychiatry 2002;59(2):131–6.

17. Kaplan GA, Seeman TE, Cohen RD, et al. Mortality among the elderly in the Alameda county study: behavioral and demographic risk factors. Am J Public Health 1987;77(3):307–12.

18. Ferrie JE, Shipley MJ, Cappuccio FP, et al. A prospective study of change in sleep duration: associations with mortality in the Whitehall II cohort. Sleep 2007;30(12):1659–66.

19. Hublin C, Partinen M, Koskenvuo M, et al. Sleep and mortality: a population-based 22-year follow-up study. Sleep 2007;30(10):1245–53.

20. Lan TY, Lan TH, Wen CP, et al. Nighttime sleep, Chinese afternoon nap, and mortality in the elderly. Sleep 2007;30(9):1105–10.

21. Gallicchio L, Kalesan B. Sleep duration and mortality: a systematic review and meta-analysis. J Sleep Res 2009;18(2):148–58.

22. Cappuccio FP, D'Elia L, Strazzullo P, et al. Sleep duration and all-cause mortality: a systematic review and meta-analysis of prospective studies. Sleep 2010;33(5):585–92.

23. Pienaar PR, Kolbe-Alexander TL, van Mechelen W, et al. Associations between self-reported sleep duration and mortality in employed individuals: systematic review and meta-analysis. Am J Health Promot 2021;35(6):853–65.

24. da Silva AA, de Mello RG, Schaan CW, et al. Sleep duration and mortality in the elderly: a systematic review with meta-analysis. BMJ Open 2016;6(2): e008119.

25. He M, Deng X, Zhu Y, et al. The relationship between sleep duration and all-cause mortality in the older people: an updated and dose-response meta-analysis. BMC Public Health 2020;20(1): 1179.

26. Liu TZ, Xu C, Rota M, et al. Sleep duration and risk of all-cause mortality: a flexible, non-linear, meta-regression of 40 prospective cohort studies. Sleep Med Rev 2017;32:28–36.

27. Khan MA, Hashim MJ, Mustafa H, et al. Global epidemiology of ischemic heart disease: results from the global burden of disease study. Cureus 2020;12(7):e9349.

28. Magee CA, Kritharides L, Attia J, et al. Short and long sleep duration are associated with prevalent cardiovascular disease in Australian adults. J Sleep Res 2012;21(4):441–7.

29. Ayas NT, White DP, Manson JE, et al. A prospective study of sleep duration and coronary heart disease in women. Arch Intern Med 2003;163(2):205–9.

30. Hoevenaar-Blom MP, Spijkerman AM, Kromhout D, et al. Sleep duration and sleep quality in relation to 12-year cardiovascular disease incidence: the MORGEN study. Sleep 2011;34(11):1487–92.

31. Aggarwal S, Loomba RS, Arora RR, et al. Associations between sleep duration and prevalence of cardiovascular events. Clin Cardiol 2013;36(11): 671–6.

32. Kwok CS, Kontopantelis E, Kuligowski G, et al. Self-reported sleep duration and quality and cardiovascular disease and mortality: a dose-response meta-analysis. J Am Heart Assoc 2018;7(15): e008552.

33. Krittanawong C, Tunhasiriwet A, Wang Z, et al. Association between short and long sleep durations and cardiovascular outcomes: a systematic review and meta-analysis. Eur Heart J Acute Cardiovasc Care 2019;8(8):762–70.

34. Cappuccio FP, Cooper D, D'Elia L, et al. Sleep duration predicts cardiovascular outcomes: a systematic review and meta-analysis of prospective studies. Eur Heart J 2011;32(12):1484–92.

35. Lao XQ, Liu X, Deng HB, et al. Sleep quality, sleep duration, and the risk of coronary heart disease: a prospective cohort study with 60,586 adults. J Clin Sleep Med 2018;14(1):109–17.

36. Chandola T, Ferrie JE, Perski A, et al. The effect of short sleep duration on coronary heart disease risk is greatest among those with sleep disturbance: a prospective study from the Whitehall II cohort. Sleep 2010;33(6):739–44.

37. Svensson AK, Svensson T, Kitlinski M, et al. Incident diabetes mellitus may explain the association

between sleep duration and incident coronary heart disease. Diabetologia 2018;61(2):331–41.

38. Chokesuwattanaskul R, Thongprayoon C, Sharma K, et al. Associations of sleep quality with incident atrial fibrillation: a meta-analysis. Intern Med J 2018;48(8):964–72.

39. Khawaja O, Sarwar A, Albert CM, et al. Sleep duration and risk of atrial fibrillation (from the Physicians' Health Study). Am J Cardiol 2013;111(4): 547–51.

40. Zhao J, Yang F, Zhuo C, et al. Association of sleep duration with atrial fibrillation and heart failure: a mendelian randomization analysis. Front Genet 2021;12:583658.

41. Morovatdar N, Ebrahimi N, Rezaee R, et al. Sleep duration and risk of atrial fibrillation: a systematic review. J Atr Fibrillation 2019;11(6):2132.

42. Mancia G, Grassi G. The autonomic nervous system and hypertension. Circ Res 2014;114(11): 1804–14.

43. Thomas SJ, Calhoun D. Sleep, insomnia, and hypertension: current findings and future directions. J Am Soc Hypertens 2017;11(2):122–9.

44. Tobaldini E, Costantino G, Solbiati M, et al. Sleep, sleep deprivation, autonomic nervous system and cardiovascular diseases. Neurosci Biobehav Rev 2017;74(Pt B):321–9.

45. Yano Y, Kario K. Nocturnal blood pressure and cardiovascular disease: a review of recent advances. Hypertens Res 2012;35(7):695–701.

46. Tochikubo O, Ikeda A, Miyajima E, et al. Effects of insufficient sleep on blood pressure monitored by a new multibiomedical recorder. Hypertension 1996; 27(6):1318–24.

47. Goncharuk VD, van Heerikhuize J, Dai JP, et al. Neuropeptide changes in the suprachiasmatic nucleus in primary hypertension indicate functional impairment of the biological clock. J Comp Neurol 2001;431(3):320–30.

48. Fang J, Wheaton AG, Keenan NL, et al. Association of sleep duration and hypertension among US adults varies by age and sex. Am J Hypertens 2012;25(3):335–41.

49. Knutson KL, Van Cauter E, Rathouz PJ, et al. Association between sleep and blood pressure in midlife: the CARDIA sleep study. Arch Intern Med 2009;169(11):1055–61.

50. Gangwisch JE, Heymsfield SB, Boden-Albala B, et al. Short sleep duration as a risk factor for hypertension: analyses of the first National Health and Nutrition Examination Survey. Hypertension 2006; 47(5):833–9.

51. Gottlieb DJ, Redline S, Nieto FJ, et al. Association of usual sleep duration with hypertension: the sleep heart health study. Sleep 2006;29(8):1009–14.

52. Wang Q, Xi B, Liu M, et al. Short sleep duration is associated with hypertension risk among adults: a systematic review and meta-analysis. Hypertens Res 2012;35(10):1012–8.

53. Shulman R, Cohen DL, Grandner MA, et al. Sleep duration and 24-hour ambulatory blood pressure in adults not on antihypertensive medications. J Clin Hypertens (Greenwich) 2018;20(12): 1712–20.

54. Cappuccio FP, Stranges S, Kandala NB, et al. Gender-specific associations of short sleep duration with prevalent and incident hypertension: the Whitehall II Study. Hypertension 2007;50(4): 693–700.

55. Li C, Shang S. Relationship between sleep and hypertension: findings from the NHANES (2007-2014). Int J Environ Res Public Health 2021; 18(15).

56. Li H, Ren Y, Wu Y, et al. Correlation between sleep duration and hypertension: a dose-response meta-analysis. J Hum Hypertens 2019;33(3):218–28.

57. Wang L, Hu Y, Wang X, et al. The association between sleep duration and hypertension: a meta and study sequential analysis. J Hum Hypertens 2021;35(7):621–6.

58. Stranges S, Dorn JM, Cappuccio FP, et al. A population-based study of reduced sleep duration and hypertension: the strongest association may be in premenopausal women. J Hypertens 2010;28(5):896–902.

59. Guo X, Zheng L, Wang J, et al. Epidemiological evidence for the link between sleep duration and high blood pressure: a systematic review and meta-analysis. Sleep Med 2013;14(4):324–32.

60. Kawada T. The definition of sleep duration and the risk for hypertension: caution for meta-analysis. Sleep Med 2013;14(12):1431.

61. McDermott M, Brown DL, Chervin RD. Sleep disorders and the risk of stroke. Expert Rev Neurother 2018;18(7):523–31.

62. Yin J, Jin X, Shan Z, et al. Relationship of sleep duration with all-cause mortality and cardiovascular events: a systematic review and dose-response meta-analysis of prospective cohort studies. J Am Heart Assoc 2017;6(9):e005947.

63. Li W, Wang D, Cao S, et al. Sleep duration and risk of stroke events and stroke mortality: a systematic review and meta-analysis of prospective cohort studies. Int J Cardiol 2016;223:870–6.

64. Cappuccio FP, Taggart FM, Kandala NB, et al. Meta-analysis of short sleep duration and obesity in children and adults. Sleep 2008;31(5):619–26.

65. Marshall NS, Glozier N, Grunstein RR. Is sleep duration related to obesity? A critical review of the epidemiological evidence. Sleep Med Rev 2008;12(4):289–98.

66. Killick R, Banks S, Liu PY. Implications of sleep restriction and recovery on metabolic outcomes. J Clin Endocrinol Metab 2012;97(11):3876–90.

67. Wu Y, Zhai L, Zhang D. Sleep duration and obesity among adults: a meta-analysis of prospective studies. Sleep Med 2014;15(12):1456–62.

68. Patel SR, Hu FB. Short sleep duration and weight gain: a systematic review. Obesity (Silver Spring) 2008;16(3):643–53.

69. Patel SR, Blackwell T, Redline S, et al. The association between sleep duration and obesity in older adults. Int J Obes (Lond) 2008;21:21.

70. Stamatakis KA, Kaplan GA, Roberts RE. Short sleep duration across income, education, and race/ethnic groups: population prevalence and growing disparities during 34 years of follow-up. Ann Epidemiol 2007;17(12):948–55.

71. Jean-Louis G, Youngstedt S, Grandner M, et al. Unequal burden of sleep-related obesity among black and white Americans. Sleep Health 2015;1(3): 169–76.

72. Zhou Q, Zhang M, Hu D. Dose-response association between sleep duration and obesity risk: a systematic review and meta-analysis of prospective cohort studies. Sleep Breath 2019;23(4):1035–45.

73. Kelly T, Yang W, Chen CS, et al. Global burden of obesity in 2005 and projections to 2030. Int J Obes (Lond) 2008;32(9):1431–7.

74. Wang Y, Beydoun MA, Liang L, et al. Will all Americans become overweight or obese? estimating the progression and cost of the US obesity epidemic. Obesity (Silver Spring) 2008;16(10):2323–30.

75. Liu B, Du Y, Wu Y, et al. Trends in obesity and adiposity measures by race or ethnicity among adults in the United States 2011-18: population based study. BMJ 2021;372:n365.

76. Simon SL, Higgins J, Melanson E, et al. A model of adolescent sleep health and risk for type 2 diabetes. Curr Diab Rep 2021;21(2):4.

77. Guo Y, Miller MA, Cappuccio FP. Short duration of sleep and incidence of overweight or obesity in Chinese children and adolescents: a systematic review and meta-analysis of prospective studies. Nutr Metab Cardiovasc Dis 2021;31(2):363–71.

78. Miller MA, Kruisbrink M, Wallace J, et al. Sleep duration and incidence of obesity in infants, children, and adolescents: a systematic review and meta-analysis of prospective studies. Sleep 2018; 41(4):zsy018.

79. Miller MA, Bates S, Ji C, et al. Systematic review and meta-analyses of the relationship between short sleep and incidence of obesity and effectiveness of sleep interventions on weight gain in preschool children. Obes Rev 2021;22(2):e13113.

80. Chaput JP, McNeil J, Despres JP, et al. Short sleep duration as a risk factor for the development of the metabolic syndrome in adults. Prev Med 2013; 57(6):872–7.

81. Hall MH, Muldoon MF, Jennings JR, et al. Self-reported sleep duration is associated with the metabolic syndrome in midlife adults. Sleep 2008; 31(5):635–43.

82. Chaput JP, McNeil J, Despres JP, et al. Seven to eight hours of sleep a night is associated with a lower prevalence of the metabolic syndrome and reduced overall cardiometabolic risk in adults. PLoS One 2013;8(9):e72832.

83. Smiley A, King D, Bidulescu A. The association between sleep duration and metabolic syndrome: the NHANES 2013/2014. Nutrients 2019;11(11):2582.

84. Kim CE, Shin S, Lee HW, et al. Association between sleep duration and metabolic syndrome: a cross-sectional study. BMC Public Health 2018;18(1): 720.

85. Stefani KM, Kim HC, Kim J, et al. The influence of sex and age on the relationship between sleep duration and metabolic syndrome in Korean adults. Diabetes Res Clin Pract 2013;102(3): 250–9.

86. Duan Y, Sun J, Wang M, et al. Association between short sleep duration and metabolic syndrome in Chinese children and adolescents. Sleep Med 2020;74:343–8.

87. Arora A, Pell D, van Sluijs EMF, et al. How do associations between sleep duration and metabolic health differ with age in the UK general population? PLoS One 2020;15(11):e0242852.

88. Xie J, Li Y, Zhang Y, et al. Sleep duration and metabolic syndrome: an updated systematic review and meta-analysis. Sleep Med Rev 2021;59:101451.

89. Hua J, Jiang H, Wang H, et al. Sleep duration and the risk of metabolic syndrome in adults: a systematic review and meta-analysis. Front Neurol 2021; 12:635564.

90. Iftikhar IH, Donley MA, Mindel J, et al. Sleep duration and metabolic syndrome. an updated dose-risk metaanalysis. Ann Am Thorac Soc 2015; 12(9):1364–72.

91. Zhao JJ, Zhang TT, Liu XH, et al. [A Meta-analysis on the association between sleep duration and metabolic syndrome in adults]. Zhonghua Liu Xing Bing Xue Za Zhi 2020;41(8):1272–9.

92. Xi B, He D, Zhang M, et al. Short sleep duration predicts risk of metabolic syndrome: a systematic review and meta-analysis. Sleep Med Rev 2014; 18(4):293–7.

93. Cappuccio FP, D'Elia L, Strazzullo P, et al. Quantity and quality of sleep and incidence of type 2 diabetes: a systematic review and meta-analysis. Diabetes Care 2010;33(2):414–20.

94. Itani O, Jike M, Watanabe N, et al. Short sleep duration and health outcomes: a systematic review, meta-analysis, and meta-regression. Sleep Med 2017;32:246–56.

95. Anothaisintawee T, Reutrakul S, Van Cauter E, et al. Sleep disturbances compared to traditional risk factors for diabetes development: systematic

review and meta-analysis. Sleep Med Rev 2016;30: 11–24.

96. Shan Z, Ma H, Xie M, et al. Sleep duration and risk of type 2 diabetes: a meta-analysis of prospective studies. Diabetes Care 2015;38(3):529–37.

97. Holliday EG, Magee CA, Kritharides L, et al. Short sleep duration is associated with risk of future diabetes but not cardiovascular disease: a prospective study and meta-analysis. PLoS One 2013; 8(11):e82305.

98. Lee SWH, Ng KY, Chin WK. The impact of sleep amount and sleep quality on glycemic control in type 2 diabetes: a systematic review and meta-analysis. Sleep Med Rev 2017;31:91–101.

99. Ji X, Wang Y, Saylor J. Sleep and type 1 diabetes mellitus management among children, adolescents, and emerging young adults: a systematic review. J Pediatr Nurs 2021;61:245–53.

100. Reutrakul S, Thakkinstian A, Anothaisintawee T, et al. Sleep characteristics in type 1 diabetes and associations with glycemic control: systematic review and meta-analysis. Sleep Med 2016;23:26–45.

101. Zhang X, Zhang R, Cheng L, et al. The effect of sleep impairment on gestational diabetes mellitus: a systematic review and meta-analysis of cohort studies. Sleep Med 2020;74:267–77.

102. Reutrakul S, Anothaisintawee T, Herring SJ, et al. Short sleep duration and hyperglycemia in pregnancy: aggregate and individual patient data meta-analysis. Sleep Med Rev 2018;40:31–42.

103. Kohansieh M, Makaryus AN. Sleep deficiency and deprivation leading to cardiovascular disease. Int J Hypertens 2015;2015:615681.

104. Carreras A, Zhang SX, Peris E, et al. Chronic Sleep fragmentation induces endothelial dysfunction and structural vascular changes in mice. Sleep 2014; 37(11):1817–24.

105. Sauvet F, Drogou C, Bougard C, et al. Vascular response to 1 week of sleep restriction in healthy subjects. A metabolic response? Int J Cardiol 2015;190:246–55.

106. Calvin AD, Covassin N, Kremers WK, et al. Experimental sleep restriction causes endothelial dysfunction in healthy humans. J Am Heart Assoc 2014;3(6):e001143.

107. Hall MH, Mulukutla S, Kline CE, et al. Objective sleep duration is prospectively associated with endothelial health. Sleep 2017;40(1):zsw003.

108. Reimund E. The free radical flux theory of sleep. Med Hypotheses 1994;43(4):231–3.

109. Atrooz F, Salim S. Sleep deprivation, oxidative stress and inflammation. Adv Protein Chem Struct Biol 2020;119:309–36.

110. Villafuerte G, Miguel-Puga A, Rodríguez EM, et al. Sleep deprivation and oxidative stress in animal models: a systematic review. Oxid Med Cell Longev 2015;2015:234952.

111. Vaccaro A, Kaplan Dor Y, Nambara K, et al. Sleep Loss can cause death through accumulation of reactive oxygen species in the gut. Cell 2020; 181(6):1307–28.e1315.

112. Jowko E, Rozanski P, Tomczak A. Effects of a 36-h survival training with sleep deprivation on oxidative stress and muscle damage biomarkers in young healthy men. Int J Environ Res Public Health 2018;15(10):2066.

113. Rozanski P, Jowko E, Tomczak A. Assessment of the levels of oxidative stress, muscle damage, and psychomotor abilities of special force soldiers during military survival training. Int J Environ Res Public Health 2020;17(13):4886.

114. Açar G, Akçakoyun M, Sari I, et al. Acute sleep deprivation in healthy adults is associated with a reduction in left atrial early diastolic strain rate. Sleep Breath 2013;17(3):975–83.

115. Cakici M, Dogan A, Cetin M, et al. Negative effects of acute sleep deprivation on left ventricular functions and cardiac repolarization in healthy young adults. Pacing Clin Electrophysiol 2015;38(6):713–22.

116. Chen WR, Shi XM, Yang TS, et al. Protective effect of metoprolol on arrhythmia and heart rate variability in healthy people with 24 hours of sleep deprivation. J Interv Card Electrophysiol 2013; 36(3):267–72 [discussion: 272].

117. Chen WH, Liu HB, Sha Y, et al. Effects of statin on arrhythmia and heart rate variability in healthy persons with 48-hour sleep deprivation. J Am Heart Assoc 2016;5(11):e003833.

118. Davies SK, Ang JE, Revell VL, et al. Effect of sleep deprivation on the human metabolome. Proc Natl Acad Sci U S A 2014;111(29):10761–6.

119. Weljie AM, Meerlo P, Goel N, et al. Oxalic acid and diacylglycerol 36:3 are cross-species markers of sleep debt. Proc Natl Acad Sci U S A 2015; 112(8):2569–74.

120. Moller-Levet CS, Archer SN, Bucca G, et al. Effects of insufficient sleep on circadian rhythmicity and expression amplitude of the human blood transcriptome. Proc Natl Acad Sci U S A 2013; 110(12):E1132–41.

121. Irwin MR, Wang M, Ribeiro D, et al. Sleep loss activates cellular inflammatory signaling. Biol Psychiatry 2008;64(6):538–40.

122. Geovanini GR, Libby P. Atherosclerosis and inflammation: overview and updates. Clin Sci (Lond) 2018;132(12):1243–52.

123. Swirski FK, Nahrendorf M. Leukocyte behavior in atherosclerosis, myocardial infarction, and heart failure. Science 2013;339(6116):161–6.

124. McAlpine CS, Kiss MG, Rattik S, et al. Sleep modulates haematopoiesis and protects against atherosclerosis. Nature 2019;566(7744):383–7.

125. Sands MR, Lauderdale DS, Liu K, et al. Short sleep duration is associated with carotid intima-media

thickness among men in the Coronary Artery Risk Development in Young Adults (CARDIA) Study. Stroke 2012;43(11):2858–64.

126. Aziz M, Ali SS, Das S, et al. Association of subjective and objective sleep duration as well as sleep quality with non-invasive markers of sub-clinical cardiovascular disease (CVD): a systematic review. J Atheroscler Thromb 2017;24(3):208–26.

127. Irwin MR, Wang M, Campomayor CO, et al. Sleep deprivation and activation of morning levels of cellular and genomic markers of inflammation. Arch Intern Med 2006;166(16):1756–62.

128. Irwin MR, Olmstead R, Carroll JE. Sleep disturbance, sleep duration, and inflammation: a systematic review and meta-analysis of cohort studies and experimental sleep deprivation. Biol Psychiatry 2016;80(1):40–52.

129. Spiegel K, Leproult R, Van Cauter E. Impact of sleep debt on metabolic and endocrine function. Lancet 1999;354(9188):1435–9.

130. Nedeltcheva AV, Kessler L, Imperial J, et al. Exposure to recurrent sleep restriction in the setting of high caloric intake and physical inactivity results in increased insulin resistance and reduced glucose tolerance. J Clin Endocrinol Metab 2009;94(9):3242–50.

131. Donga E, van Dijk M, van Dijk JG, et al. A single night of partial sleep deprivation induces insulin resistance in multiple metabolic pathways in healthy subjects. J Clin Endocrinol Metab 2010;95(6):2963–8.

132. Zielinski MR, Kline CE, Kripke DF, et al. No effect of 8-week time in bed restriction on glucose tolerance in older long sleepers. J Sleep Res 2008;5:5.

133. van Leeuwen WM, Hublin C, Sallinen M, et al. Prolonged sleep restriction affects glucose metabolism in healthy young men. Int J Endocrinol 2010;2010:108641.

134. Bosy-Westphal A, Hinrichs S, Jauch-Chara K, et al. Influence of partial sleep deprivation on energy balance and insulin sensitivity in healthy women. Obes Facts 2008;1(5):266–73.

135. Schmid SM, Jauch-Chara K, Hallschmid M, et al. Mild sleep restriction acutely reduces plasma glucagon levels in healthy men. J Clin Endocrinol Metab 2009;94(12):5169–73.

136. Buxton OM, Pavlova M, Reid EW, et al. Sleep restriction for 1 week reduces insulin sensitivity in healthy men. Diabetes 2010;59(9):2126–33.

137. St-Onge MP, O'Keeffe M, Roberts AL, et al. Short sleep duration, glucose dysregulation and hormonal regulation of appetite in men and women. Sleep 2012;35(11):1503–10.

138. Morselli LL, Guyon A, Spiegel K. Sleep and metabolic function. Pflugers Archiv 2012;463(1):139–60.

139. Morselli L, Leproult R, Balbo M, et al. Role of sleep duration in the regulation of glucose metabolism and appetite. Best Pract Res Clin Endocrinol Metab 2010;24(5):687–702.

140. Killick R, Hoyos CM, Melehan K, et al. Metabolic and hormonal effects of 'catch-up' sleep in men with chronic, repetitive, lifestyle-driven sleep restriction. Clin Endocrinol (Oxf) 2015;83(4):498–507.

141. Markwald RR, Melanson EL, Smith MR, et al. Impact of insufficient sleep on total daily energy expenditure, food intake, and weight gain. Proc Natl Acad Sci U S A 2013;110(14):5695–700.

142. Shechter A, Rising R, Albu JB, et al. Experimental sleep curtailment causes wake-dependent increases in 24-h energy expenditure as measured by whole-room indirect calorimetry. Am J Clin Nutr 2013;98(6):1433–9.

143. St-Onge MP, Roberts AL, Chen J, et al. Short sleep duration increases energy intakes but does not change energy expenditure in normal-weight individuals. Am J Clin Nutr 2011;94(2):410–6.

144. Spaeth AM, Dinges DF, Goel N. Effects of experimental sleep restriction on weight gain, caloric intake, and meal timing in healthy adults. Sleep 2013;36(7):981–90.

145. Capers PL, Fobian AD, Kaiser KA, et al. A systematic review and meta-analysis of randomized controlled trials of the impact of sleep duration on adiposity and components of energy balance. Obes Rev 2015;16(9):771–82.

146. Al Khatib HK, Harding SV, Darzi J, et al. The effects of partial sleep deprivation on energy balance: a systematic review and meta-analysis. Eur J Clin Nutr 2017;71(5):614–24.

147. Gallegos JV, Boege HL, Zuraikat FM, et al. Does sex influence the effects of experimental sleep curtailment and circadian misalignment on regulation of appetite? Curr Opin Endocr Metab Res 2021;17:20–5.

148. McNeil J, St-Onge MP. Increased energy intake following sleep restriction in men and women: a one-size-fits-all conclusion? Obesity (Silver Spring) 2017;25(6):989–92.

149. St-Onge MP, McReynolds A, Trivedi ZB, et al. Sleep restriction leads to increased activation of brain regions sensitive to food stimuli. Am J Clin Nutr 2012;95(4):818–24.

150. St-Onge MP, Wolfe S, Sy M, et al. Sleep restriction increases the neuronal response to unhealthy food in normal-weight individuals. Int J Obes (Lond) 2014;38(3):411–6.

151. Hoddy KK, Potts KS, Bazzano LA, et al. Sleep extension: a potential target for obesity treatment. Curr Diab Rep 2020;20(12):81.

152. Zhu B, Yin Y, Shi C, et al. Feasibility of sleep extension and its effect on cardiometabolic parameters in free-living settings: a systematic review and meta-analysis of experimental studies. Eur J Cardiovasc Nurs 2022;21(1):9–25.

153. Pizinger TM, Aggarwal B, St-Onge MP. Sleep extension in short sleepers: an evaluation of feasibility and effectiveness for weight management and cardiometabolic disease prevention. Front Endocrinol (Lausanne) 2018;9:392.

154. Kothari V, Cardona Z, Chirakalwasan N, et al. Sleep interventions and glucose metabolism: systematic review and meta-analysis. Sleep Med 2021;78: 24–35.

155. Henst RHP, Pienaar PR, Roden LC, et al. The effects of sleep extension on cardiometabolic risk factors: a systematic review. J Sleep Res 2019; 28(6):e12865.

156. Al Khatib HK, Hall WL, Creedon A, et al. Sleep extension is a feasible lifestyle intervention in free-living adults who are habitually short sleepers: a potential strategy for decreasing intake of free sugars? A randomized controlled pilot study. Am J Clin Nutr 2018;107(1):43–53.

157. So-Ngern A, Chirakalwasan N, Saetung S, et al. Effects of two-week sleep extension on glucose metabolism in chronically sleep-deprived individuals. J Clin Sleep Med 2019;15(5):711–8.

158. Reutrakul S, So-Ngern A, Chirakalwasan N, et al. No changes in gut microbiota after two-week sleep extension in chronically sleep-deprived individuals. Sleep Med 2020;68:27–30.

159. Stock AA, Lee S, Nahmod NG, et al. Effects of sleep extension on sleep duration, sleepiness, and blood pressure in college students. Sleep Health 2020;6(1):32–9.

160. Tasali E, Chapotot F, Wroblewski K, et al. The effects of extended bedtimes on sleep duration and food desire in overweight young adults: a home-based intervention. Appetite 2014;80:220–4.

161. Leproult R, Deliens G, Gilson M, et al. Beneficial impact of sleep extension on fasting insulin sensitivity in adults with habitual sleep restriction. Sleep 2015;38(5):707–15.

162. Haack M, Serrador J, Cohen D, et al. Increasing sleep duration to lower beat-to-beat blood pressure: a pilot study. J Sleep Res 2013;22(3): 295–304.

163. Reynold AM, Bowles ER, Saxena A, et al. Negative effects of time in bed extension: a pilot study. J Sleep Med Disord 2014;1(1):1002.

164. Baron KG, Duffecy J, Richardson D, et al. Technology assisted behavior intervention to extend sleep among adults with short sleep duration and prehypertension/stage 1 hypertension: a randomized pilot feasibility study. J Clin Sleep Med 2019;15(11): 1587–97.

165. Moreno-Frias C, Figueroa-Vega N, Malacara JM. Sleep extension increases the effect of caloric restriction over body weight and improves the chronic low-grade inflammation in adolescents with obesity. J Adolesc Health 2020;66(5): 575–81.

166. Hartescu I, Stensel DJ, Thackray AE, et al. Sleep extension and metabolic health in male overweight/obese short sleepers: a randomised controlled trial. J Sleep Res 2022;31(2):e13469.

Assessment of Vigilance and Fatigue

Tyler Johnson, MD[a],*, Indira Gurubhagavatula, MD[a,b],**

KEYWORDS

- Vigilance • Fatigue • Sleepiness • Epworth sleepiness scale (ESS)
- Stanford sleepiness scale (SSS) • Karolinska sleepiness scale (KSS)
- Multiple sleep latency test (MSLT) • Maintenance of wakefulness test (MWT)

KEY POINTS

- Vigilance, fatigue, and sleepiness are distinct clinical entities.
- Various subjective and objective tests have been developed in order to diagnose and quantify each entity.
- More research is needed to develop more accurate and cost-effective tools for diagnosis.

INTRODUCTION

Although often used interchangeably, fatigue, sleepiness, and vigilance are distinct entities. Differentiating among them is necessary in order to address performance, health, and safety. Self-reported fatigue is common and experienced by 7.6% to 41.2% of the population.[1–3] In sleep centers, sleepiness may be the presenting complaint in 16% to 33% or more of patients.[4,5] From a public health perspective, fatigue and sleepiness can have profound influence on safety: some 16.5% of fatal vehicular crashes, for example, have been attributed to drowsy driving.[6,7] Furthermore, a recent meta-analysis suggested sleepiness while driving significantly increased the risk of motor vehicle accidents (pooled odds ratio [OR] 2.51; 95% confidence interval [CI] 1.87–3.39).[8] In the workplace, sleepiness has been linked with safety incidents and errors (including catastrophic events, such as the Space Shuttle Challenger, Chernobyl, and Exxon Valdez disasters), absenteeism, presenteeism, and occupational burnout.[9–11] Health effects of chronic sleepiness may include errors in judgment, obesity, hypertension, cardiovascular

disease, hyperlipidemia, type 2 diabetes mellitus, and mood disorders, among others.[11–13] In this text, we will explore common methods used to assess sleepiness, fatigue, and vigilance, and summarize recent technological advances in measurement approaches.

DEFINITIONS

Fatigue is often used interchangeably with sleepiness in operational settings, such as workplaces where safety-sensitive work is being performed. In clinical settings, however, fatigue and sleepiness are distinct, with fatigue referring to physical rather than mental tiredness. For example, anemia, cancer chemotherapy, or the use of beta-blockers may contribute to a sense of physical fatigue. In operational settings, however, in addition to physical fatigue, the concept of mental fatigue is also recognized. Perception of fatigue, thus, may be defined as a subjective sensation of tiredness and reduced capacity for performance or exertion in either the physical or mental domains.[14,15] Sleepiness, however, is most often defined as the propensity for a subject to fall

a Division of Sleep Medicine, Perelman School of Medicine, University of Pennsylvania, 3624 Market Street, Suite 205, Philadelphia, PA 19104, USA; b Crescenz VA Medical Center, Philadelphia, PA, USA
* Corresponding author.
** Corresponding author. Division of Sleep Medicine, Perelman School of Medicine, University of Pennsylvania, 3624 Market Street, Suite 205, Philadelphia, PA 19104, USA
E-mail addresses: Tyler.Johnson@pennmedicine.upenn.edu; tjj4k@virginia.edu (T.J.); Indira@pennmedicine.upenn.edu (I.G.)

Sleep Med Clin 18 (2023) 349–359
https://doi.org/10.1016/j.jsmc.2023.05.007

asleep in a situation when normally expected to be awake or alert.[16] Van Schie and colleagues recently defined vigilance as "the capability to be aware of relevant, unpredictable changes in one's environment, irrespective of whether or not such changes occur." Vigilance may be quantified in 2 dimensions—the level of alertness required to complete a task and how it can change over time.[17]

SUBJECTIVE ASSESSMENT OF SLEEPINESS

Both subjective and objective validated tools are available for assessing sleepiness. Subjective tests include the Epworth Sleepiness Scale (ESS), Stanford Sleepiness Scale (SSS), and Karolinska Sleepiness Scale (KSS), whereas objective tests include the multiple sleep latency test (MSLT), the maintenance of wakefulness test (MWT), and a less-commonly used variation of the MWT known as the Oxford Sleep Resistance (OSLER) test. Other tests with less-established roles in the clinical evaluation of sleepiness include pupillometry, evoked potential monitoring, and the alpha attenuation test. This section will discuss the strengths and limitations of these strategies.

Epworth Sleepiness Scale

The ESS is one of the most commonly used subjective screening tools.[18] Developed and validated by Dr Murray Johns in 1991, the ESS is an 8-item questionnaire that asks subjects to rate "how likely [they] are to doze off or fall asleep, in contrast to just feeling tired" during each of 8 sedentary situations on a scale of 0 to 3 (0 being no chance of dozing; 3 being a high chance). Subjects are told to select their scores based on experience in their "usual way of life in recent times." Therefore, the score is a summative, subjective evaluation of sleepiness during a period of weeks. Scores range from 0 to 24, with a score greater than 10 indicating "pathological sleepiness" (**Fig. 1**).[19] The ESS has been validated in numerous populations, including patients with stroke, epilepsy, and

Parkinson disease, as well as pediatric patients aged as young as 7 years (Epworth Sleepiness Scale for Children and Adolescents).[20–23] Developed originally in English, the ESS has been translated and validated in Arabic, Spanish, French, Mandarin, Hindi, Portuguese, and other languages.[24–29] The ESS has been shown to have substantial test–retest reliability with classification into normal (ESS 10 or less) versus sleepy (ESS 11 or greater).[30,31] Advantages of the ESS include its speed, ease of use, convenience, minimal training requirement, and ability to be self-administered. Limitations of the ESS include some intraindividual variability because variation in score can occur if tested day-to-day. Additionally, the ESS is less effective in capturing immediate-term sleepiness—an attribute much better assessed with the SSS.[32] Moreover, subjects with cognitive limitation may have difficulty with multistep instructions, such as "even if you have not done some of these things recently, try to determine how they would have affected you."

Stanford Sleepiness Scale

The SSS is another validated subjective measure of sleepiness. First described by Hoddes, Dement, and Zarcone in the early 1970s, the SSS is designed to quantify progressive changes in sleepiness.[33] At any point in time, subjects are asked to rate their sleepiness on a scale of 1 to 7 (**Fig. 2**).[34] The SSS is more suitable for assessing sleepiness due to acute sleep deprivation than the ESS and is able to quantify changes in sleepiness within short period but is less able to differentiate sleep-deprived normal subjects from those with chronic sleep disorders.[35] Furthermore, subjects with untreated sleep disorders such as sleep apnea have been shown to have sizable discordances between SSS scores and behavioral indicators of sleep. For example, subjects may record "normal" SSS scores while exhibiting closed eyes and snoring.[36] Thus, the SSS is used more commonly in research than clinical practice, most often as a measurement of the

Epworth Sleepiness Scale				
Rate the following situations how likely you are to doze off or fall asleep, in contrast to just feeling tired.				
Even if you have not done some of these things recently, try to determine how they would have affected you				
Scale: 0 = No chance of dozing; 1 = Slight chance of dozing; 2 = Moderate chance of dozing; 3 = High chance of dozing				
Sitting and reading	0	1	2	3
Watching television	0	1	2	3
Sitting inactive in a public place	0	1	2	3
Riding as a passenger in a car for 1 h without a break	0	1	2	3
Lying down to rest in the afternoon when circumstances permit	0	1	2	3
Sitting and talking with someone	0	1	2	3
Sitting quietly after lunch without alcohol	0	1	2	3
Sitting in a car as the driver while stopped for a few minutes in traffic	0	1	2	3
Total ____ /24 (>10 considered pathologically sleepy)				

Fig. 1. The ESS: A validated, subjective scale for the evaluation of sleepiness. (*Data from*: Johns MW. A new method for measuring daytime sleepiness: the Epworth sleepiness scale. Sleep. 1991;14(6):540-545. https://doi.org/10.1093/sleep/14.6.540.)

Stanford Sleepiness Scale	
Select the one number that best describes your level of alertness or sleepiness right now	
Degree of sleepiness	**Rating**
Feeling active, vital, alert, or wide awake	1
Functioning at high levels, but not at peak; able to concentrate	2
Awake, but relaxed; responsive but not fully alert	3
Somewhat foggy, let down	4
Foggy; losing interest in remaining awake; slowed down	5
Sleepy, woozy, fighting sleep; prefer to lie down	6
No longer fighting sleep, sleep onset soon; losing struggle to remain awake	7

Fig. 2. The SSS: A validated, subjective scale for the measurement of sleepiness. (*Data from*: Hoddes, E, Dement W, Zarcone V. The history and use of the Stanford Sleepiness Scale. Psychophysiology, 1972, 9, 150.)

impact of acute sleep loss on immediately perceived subjective sleepiness.

Karolinska Sleepiness Scale

Similar to the SSS, the KSS is designed to measure the subjective amount of sleepiness a patient experiences at a particular time. Subjects are asked to indicate their alertness/sleepiness on a 9-point scale (as opposed to the 7-point scale of the SSS), based on how they felt during the last 5 minutes (**Fig. 3**).[37] Studies have validated the KSS against alpha and theta electroencephalographic (EEG) activity, and have also demonstrated that falling asleep at the wheel in a diving simulator was preceded by an increase in KSS score.[38–40] Similar to the SSS, the KSS is primarily a tool used in research studies to evaluate acute sleepiness in various scenarios, such as studies of shift work, jet lag, driving abilities, attention, and performance.[41–46]

OBJECTIVE ASSESSMENT OF SLEEPINESS
Multiple Sleep Latency Test

The MSLT is an objective measure of sleepiness designed to test how quickly a subject falls asleep in a controlled environment during a series of nap opportunities.[47] First described by Mary Carskadon and William Dement in the 1970s, the MSLT is considered the "gold standard" measurement

of sleepiness.[48] Due to its high sensitivity and reproducibility, the MSLT is the most commonly used objective test of sleepiness in clinical settings.[49] The typical indication is to diagnose narcolepsy or idiopathic hypersomnia but the MSLT is sensitive in detecting sleepiness from other causes as well, including sedating medications, insufficient sleep, and sleep apnea. To improve specificity, testing facilities must follow a strict protocol defined by the American Academy of Sleep Medicine (AASM), most recently revised in 2021. For at least 2 weeks before testing, patients should obtain adequate sleep with a regular sleep–wake schedule, which ideally can be recorded using a sleep diary or actigraphy. Obstructive sleep apnea (OSA) and other sleep disorders should also be excluded or well treated before the MSLT. Positive airway pressure (PAP) or non-PAP therapies such as hypoglossal nerve stimulation for those with OSA should be continued during the polysomnogram (PSG) the night before the MSLT, as well as during the MSLT itself (a change reflected in the revised 2021 AASM MSLT/MWT protocols based on the theoretical concern that inadequately treated OSA could lead to a false-positive MSLT). Alerting, sedating, rapid eye movement (REM)-sleep-suppressing medications, and caffeine should be discontinued before the MSLT, with a taper if necessary to avoid withdrawal symptoms.[50]

The MSLT consists of 5 nap trials at 2-hour intervals. The patient begins each trial lying in bed in a dark, comfortable room and is given the instructions: "Please lie quietly, assume a comfortable position, keep your eyes closed, and allow yourself to fall asleep." Each trial is ended within 20 minutes if the patient does not fall asleep, as measured by frontal, central, and occipital EEG (at least one recording lead for each site). If the patient does fall asleep, the trial is continued for an additional 15 minutes. Between nap trials, the patient must be out of bed and should not be permitted to sleep; however, exposure to bright light, vigorous exercise, or stimulants must be avoided. Furthermore, the MSLT should only be performed after an attended PSG the previous night, which

Karolinska Sleepiness Scale	
Please rate your sleepiness over the past 5 min	
Extremely alert	1
Very alert	2
Alert	3
Rather alert	4
Neither alert nor sleepy	5
Some signs of sleepiness	6
Sleepy but no effort to keep awake	7
Sleepy but some effort to keep awake	8
Very sleepy with great effort to keep awake	9

Fig. 3. Karolinska Sleepiness Scale: The KSS is a validated subjective measure of sleepiness. (*Data from*: Akerstedt T, Gillberg M. Subjective and objective sleepiness in the active individual. Int J Neurosci. 1990;52(1-2):29-37. https://doi.org/10.3109/00207459008994241.)

demonstrated at least 6 hours of sleep and 7 hours in bed (PAP pressures should not be adjusted during the PSG). Sleep latency is defined as the time from lights out until the start of the first epoch of sleep; if no sleep occurs during the nap trial, the sleep latency is 20 minutes for that nap trial.[50]

In the interpretation of the MSLT, abnormal mean sleep latency is defined as less than or equal to 8 minutes; if accompanied by 2 or more sleep onset REM periods (SOREMPs), the findings are consistent with narcolepsy (a mean sleep onset latency of less than 8 minutes without 2 SOREMPs would be consistent with idiopathic hypersomnia).[50] However, the test results must be interpreted with caution, particularly in shift workers and those with sleep deprivation. The Wisconsin Sleep Cohort found that shift workers were 4 to 7 times more likely to have 2 or more SOREMPs than nonshift workers.[51] Furthermore, the same study demonstrated lack of stability of MSLT findings at a 4-year interval, even after accounting for confounding variables such as shift work.[51] Due to this lack of specificity, the MSLT alone should not be the sole criteria for diagnosing the cause of excessive sleepiness; other clinical findings are critically important for confirming a diagnosis of narcolepsy or idiopathic hypersomnia.

Some limitations of the MSLT include lack of establishment of "normal" values because sleep latencies can vary widely between healthy individuals, as well as the same individual at different ages. Chronic insomnia may also influence sleep latency. Another source of confounding may be the inability to discontinue medications before the MSLT (particularly REM-suppressing medications); alternatively, abrupt discontinuation of these medications before testing may lead to false-positive results due to rebound REM sleep.[52] Additional studies are needed to define normal sleep latency in various groups and to elucidate the influence of factors such as age; sleep timing; hormonal cycles; sleep disorders such as shift work, other medical disorders, chronic pain; and the use of recreational drugs such as marijuana on test results.[50] Other limitations include high expense, requirement for prolonged time and technical expertise, and dependence on a laboratory setting.[53–58]

Maintenance of Wakefulness Test

Although the MSLT measures tendency to fall asleep, the MWT is a validated, objective assessment of alertness/ability to stay awake. Although less commonly performed clinically than the MSLT, the MWT can be performed to help determine the patient's ability to stay awake compared with normal controls. It can also be used to determine the effect of interventions (such as stimulants) on a patient's ability to stay awake.[50]

The MWT consists of four 40-minute wake trials at 2-hour intervals, with the initial trial beginning 90 to 180 minutes after the patient wakes up from the previous night's sleep. Unlike the MSLT, a preceding PSG is not necessary for the MWT, although it may be useful if a sleep disorder such as obstructive sleep apnea is suspected. Moreover, unlike the MSLT, patients are generally continued on any stimulants or pharmacotherapy before the test because the MWT is often used to determine response to therapy. Patients should be monitored with the same EEG/audiovisual recording used in the MSLT and be seated in a bed or reclining chair with the back and head supported for each wake trial. The room should be dimly lit with a light source of 0.1 to 0.13 lux at the corneal level, placed 12 inches off the floor and 3 feet lateral to the patient's head. Immediately before the start of the wake trial, the patient should be instructed: "Please sit still and remain awake for as long as possible. Look directly ahead of you, and do not look directly at the light." Each wake trial is terminated after 3 consecutive epochs (30-second intervals) of N1 sleep, any epoch of any sleep stage that is not N1, or after 40 minutes has elapsed, with mean sleep latency averaged over the 4 trials (if no sleep occurred during a trial, 40 minutes is used for the calculation of mean sleep latency). Similar to the MSLT, the MWT must be interpreted by a board eligible or board certified sleep medicine physician.[50]

Normal values for the MWT are not well-defined. Previous studies have indicated normal mean sleep latency to be 30.4 ± 11.2 minutes on the MWT, with abnormal values to be less than 12.9 minutes or 16.1 minutes.[59–61] One recent study supports that motor vehicle accident risk increases 5-fold in patients unable to stay awake longer than 19 minutes on an average versus those able to stay awake for an average of 33 minutes or longer.[62] Similar to the MSLT, limitations of the MWT include long duration, high cost, need for a sleep medicine specialist, and appropriate clinical context for accurate interpretation. Future studies are needed to better elucidate the impact of MWT findings on performance in various settings.

Oxford Sleep Resistance Test

The OSLER test is a derivation of the MWT where onset of sleep is determined by the failure to perform a certain action rather than EEG criteria. Similar to the MWT, an individual undergoes four 40-minute sleep challenges at 2-hour intervals during the course of the day. During those wake trials, the patient is asked to press a switch in response to a light-emitting diode (LED) screen, which flashes light every 3 seconds. Sleep is defined when 7 consecutive light flashes occur without the patient pressing the switch.[63] The OSLER test has the advantage of being less expensive, less labor intensive, and easier to administer than the MWT, and has a sensitivity and specificity of detecting sleep (greater than or equal to 3 seconds in duration) of 85% and 94%, respectively.[64] Derivations of the OSLER test also exist, including a portable, shorter version called the TRES test (Spanish acronym for Test de REsistencia al Sueño), where a single 20-minute session is used between 9 AM and 11 AM and subjects are asked to pass their finger over a groove in response to seeing a flash of light emanating from LED-emitting glasses.[65] Despite being simpler and less expensive than the MWT, the OSLER test is rarely used clinically, and requires further study in order to better establish normative values.

Pupillometry

Pupillometry has been available since the 1950s, when investigators recognized that certain variable characteristics of the pupillary reflex may be related to sleepiness/wakefulness due to alterations in the autonomic nervous system with sleep deprivation.[66–68] During pupillometry, patients are asked to fixate on a red target over 15 minutes while remaining awake in a darkened room. An infrared pupillometer measures pupil diameter at intervals. Calculated metrics, including the ratio of the mean pupil diameter in any given interval to the mean diameter during the first interval, the pupillary unrest index, and the energy of pupil movement in different frequency bands, have correlated to various degrees with MSLT sleep onset latency.[69] Another metric is percent eyelid closure over the pupil in drivers using a dashboard-mounted device.[70] The pupillographic sleepiness test has been evaluated in fitness-for-duty or fitness-to-drive testing at test durations ranging from 82 seconds to 11 minutes. One report demonstrated that 5.5 minutes was the shortest test duration where accuracy remained high across different types of impairment.[71] Despite its convenience, the clinical and commercial use of pupillometry remains limited due to high cost, complexity, and limited range of applicability.[16] Efforts are underway, however, to develop less-expensive application-based pupillometry with improved accuracy, which eventually could be appropriate for commercial use.[72]

Evoked Potential Monitoring

Data show that cortical and visual/auditory-evoked potentials can have long latency in states of sleepiness and with sleep disorders such as narcolepsy and OSA.[16] However, their clinical use remains limited due to high degrees of inter-subject variability, expense, and need for technical proficiency.[73]

Alpha Attenuation Test

As individuals transition from being alert to sleepy, the alpha frequency (8–12 Hz) range decreases to the theta (4–8 Hz).[74] During the alpha attenuation test, subjects are instructed to open and close their eyes 8 times, with each opening and closing lasting for 1 minute (although variations of this protocol have been described).[16,74] Various studies have shown that the ratio of mean eyes closed to mean eyes open power differs significantly between patients with excessive sleepiness (such as narcoleptics) compared with controls.[74,75] However, practical/clinical application is limited by the need for complex EEG monitoring, time, and expense.

ASSESSMENT OF FATIGUE

Unlike sleepiness, objective measures of fatigue are still unavailable, and this metric can only be measured subjectively. Fatigue is nonetheless confused with sleepiness because overlap between the 2 is common. Fatigue refers to the subjective sensation of tiredness and reduced capacity for physical or mental exertion.[14] Fatigue may also be categorized as acute, chronic, physiological, psychological, central, and peripheral.[16] Many subjective tools have been developed to measure fatigue: the fatigue severity scale (FSS), the fatigue impact scale (FIS), the fatigue questionnaire, the fatigue assessment instrument, the multidimensional fatigue inventory, the brief fatigue inventory, the Chalder fatigue scale, and the visual analog scale for fatigue, to name a few. The most commonly used of these tools, the FSS and FIS, will be discussed below.

Fatigue Severity Scale

Perhaps the best-known and most used scale for the quantification of fatigue is the FSS. The FSS is a 9-item scale that measures the impact of fatigue on specific types of functioning. Subjects are asked to rate 9 statements on level of agreement or disagreement, with a rating of one indicating strong disagreement, and a rating of 7 indicating strong agreement (**Fig. 4**).[76] The FSS has good test–retest reliability with high internal

Fatigue Severity Scale

Please choose a number between 1 and 7 that indicates your degree of agreement with the following statements. 1 indicates strongly disagree and 7 indicates strongly agree.

1. My motivation is lower when I am fatigued		1 2 3 4 5 6 7
2. Exercise brings on my fatigue		1 2 3 4 5 6 7
3. I am easily fatigued		1 2 3 4 5 6 7
4. Fatigue interferes with my physical functioning		1 2 3 4 5 6 7
5. Fatigue causes frequent problems for me		1 2 3 4 5 6 7
6. My fatigue prevents sustained physical functioning		1 2 3 4 5 6 7
7. Fatigue interferes with carrying out certain duties and responsibilities		1 2 3 4 5 6 7
8. Fatigue is among my three most disabling symptoms		1 2 3 4 5 6 7
9. Fatigue interferes with my work, family, or social life		1 2 3 4 5 6 7

Fig. 4. The FSS: A validated subjective measurement of fatigue. The sum of the 9 statements is divided by 9 to produce an average score among all responses. (*Data from*: Krupp LB, LaRocca NG, Muir-Nash J, Steinberg AD. The fatigue severity scale. Application to patients with multiple sclerosis and systemic lupus erythematosus. Arch Neurol. 1989;46(10):1121-1123. https://doi.org/10.1001/archneur.1989.00520460115022.)

consistency, is sensitive to change with time and treatment, and shows differential findings in different disease states, such as chronic fatigue syndrome/myalgic encephalomyelitis, multiple sclerosis, systemic lupus erythematosus, and primary depression.[76–78] It is also short and able to be completed quickly, even in patients suffering from significant fatigue.

Fatigue Impact Scale

The FIS is a 40-item questionnaire, which assesses the impact of fatigue on cognitive, physical, or psychosocial functioning. The FIS was originally validated in patients with multiple sclerosis and chronic hypertension, and has been validated in other populations since then.[79,80] Its limitations include the length of the questionnaire, which may pose a particular challenge for fatigued individuals.[81] A contemporary 21-item Modified Fatigue Impact Scale (MFIS) has also been validated in multiple sclerosis patients and is often utilized because of its shorter length (**Fig. 5**).[82,83]

ASSESSMENT OF VIGILANCE

Van Schie and colleagues proposed a definition of vigilance as "the capability to be aware of relevant, unpredictable changes in one's environment,

Modified Fatigue Impact Scale

Below is a list of statements that describe how fatigue may affect a person. Fatigue is a feeling of physical tiredness and lack of energy that many people experience from time to time. Please read each statement carefully, then circle the one number that best indicates how often fatigue has affected you in this way during the past 4 wk.

	Never	Rarely	Sometimes	Often	Almost Always
1. I have been less alert	0	1	2	3	4
2. I have had difficulty paying attention for long periods of time	0	1	2	3	4
3. I have been unable to think clearly	0	1	2	3	4
4. I have been clumsy and uncoordinated	0	1	2	3	4
5. I have been forgetful	0	1	2	3	4
6. I have had to pace myself in my physical activities	0	1	2	3	4
7. I have been less motivated to do anything that requires physical effort	0	1	2	3	4
8. I have been less motivated to participate in social activities	0	1	2	3	4
9. I have been less motivated to do things away from home	0	1	2	3	4
10. I have had trouble maintaining physical effort for long periods	0	1	2	3	4
11. I have had difficulty making decisions	0	1	2	3	4
12. I have been less motivated to do anything that requires thinking	0	1	2	3	4
13. My muscles have felt weak	0	1	2	3	4
14. I have been physically uncomfortable	0	1	2	3	4
15. I have had trouble finishing tasks that require thinking	0	1	2	3	4
16. I have had difficulty organizing my thoughts when doing things at home or work	0	1	2	3	4
17. I have been less able to complete tasks that require physical effort	0	1	2	3	4
18. My thinking has been slowed down	0	1	2	3	4
19. I have had trouble concentrating	0	1	2	3	4
20. I have limited my physical activities	0	1	2	3	4
21. I have needed to rest more often or for longer periods	0	1	2	3	4

Fig. 5. The MFIS: A validated scale for the evaluation of fatigue, which is often used in multiple sclerosis patients. Items can be aggregated into 3 subscales: physical, cognitive, and psychosocial, as well as into a total MFIS score. Physical subscale: 0 to 36. Computed by adding raw scores on #4, #6, #7, #10, #13, #14, #17, #20, #21 Cognitive subscale: 0 to 40. Computed by adding raw scores on #1, #2, #3, #5, #11, #12, #15, #16, #18, #19 Psychosocial subscale: 0 to 8. Computed by adding raw scores on #8 and #9. Total MFIS score: 0 to 84 (38 is often used as a cutoff for fatigue). (*Data from*: Kos D, Kerckhofs E, Carrea I, Verza R, Ramos M, Jansa J. Evaluation of the Modified Fatigue Impact Scale in four different European countries. Mult Scler. 2005;11:76–80.)

irrespective of whether or not such changes occur."[17] Thus, there is significant overlap in the evaluation of sleepiness and vigilance, although the 2 entities may be considered conceptual opposites. The primary tool to assess vigilance is the psychomotor vigilance test (PVT). However, although less commonly used than the PVT, other tests such as the divided attention driving test (DADT) have been shown to strongly correlate with the PVT and may be more applicable to specific high-risk scenarios such as drowsy driving.[18] Finally, tests such as the sustained attention to response task (SART) may be applicable to high-stakes scenarios such as whether or not to pull the trigger in a combat situation.[84]

Psychomotor Vigilance Test

The PVT is a test of sustained attention, measuring the speed at which individuals respond to visual stimuli. The test requires participants to rapidly respond to visual cues presented within specified interstimulus intervals. Subjects were asked to press a button as soon as they see a light appear on a screen, with the light turning on at random intervals during a 3 or 10-minute test.[85,86] Response times are recorded and evaluated. Sleep deprivation is known to cause an overall slowing of response time (defined as response times ≥ 500 milliseconds), an increase in the number of errors of omission (lapses), and an increase in responses without a stimulus (errors of commission).[83] The PVT is considered the gold-standard measure of deficits encountered with sleep loss and is the most commonly used test to assess vigilance in clinical research.[87]

Divided Attention Driving Test

Originally described by George and colleagues in 1996, the DADT is a 20-minute test performed on a computer-based driving simulator. Subjects are asked to steer a cursor within 2 lines on the computer screen (designed to represent lane boundaries), which are continuously moved side-to-side in random amounts (to represent the task of staying in a lane while driving). This represents "tracking" ability. While "steering" the cursor, the numbers 0 to 9 appear at random intervals in the corners of the screen—in the most common version of the test, subjects are asked to press a button on the same side of the steering wheel when the number "2" appears in a corner of the screen. This task represents "visual search."[88] When mean tracking error is defined as the primary outcome, the DADT has been shown to correlate with other measures of vigilance and sleepiness, such as the PVT and MSLT.[18] However, the DADT is not used as

commonly as the PVT, likely due to higher cost and the need for more specialized equipment.

Sustained Attention to Response Task

Sleepiness can manifest as the inability to sustain attention for a prolonged period, therefore resulting in the commission of mistakes or complete lapses when attending to a task. Originally described by Robertson and colleagues in 1997, the SART is a task in which errors of *commission* are used to assess sustained attention, as opposed to errors of *omission*.[89] In the SART, subjects are coached to respond to a "Go" stimulus, whereas withholding response to a "No-Go" stimulus. Although there are slight variations, the task is roughly 4.3 minutes in length and consists of approximately 225 trials; during each trial, a digit appears for 250 milliseconds with an interval of 900 ms between consecutive digits. Participants are instructed to press a keyboard key as soon as possible to all digits that appear ("Go" stimuli) except for "3," to which they are instructed to withhold response ("No-Go" stimulus).[84] Response time is recorded, as well as errors of commission (inappropriately responding to "No-Go" stimulus) and errors of omission (not responding to "Go" stimulus).[90] The SART assesses the "speed-accuracy trade-off" and thus has the applicability in the evaluation of patients with traumatic brain injury and neurodegenerative disease, as well as in tasks such as the direction of automated systems, combat engagement, use of force encounters by police, and security screening.[84,91–93]

SUMMARY

Sleepiness, fatigue, and vigilance are highly clinically relevant, particularly in the field of sleep medicine. Results of testing can suggest specific diagnoses, such as narcolepsy and idiopathic hypersomnia, and also hold clinical relevance for performance, particularly in critical tasks such as driving, boating, aviation, and patient care. These represent serious public health concerns, as noted extensively in the literature.[94–97] Burnout is also an important consideration in chronic sufferers, and represents great personal and taxpayer/commercial cost.[98–102] Many of the methods of assessing sleepiness, fatigue, and vigilance are not ideal, either due to subjectivity, incomplete understanding, and/or the high cost, time commitment, and training necessary to conduct them appropriately. There is also some disagreement regarding the exact definitions of each of these terms.[103] Additional research and development is necessary in order to develop newer, objective methods that are more applicable in different scenarios.

CLINICS CARE POINTS

- Fatigue, sleepiness, and the ability to remain vigilant represent important public health concerns.

- Current tools used in the assessment of fatigue, sleepiness, and vigilance are often overly subjective; many of the objective tools being developed require further validation and/ or are difficult to implement clinically (due to high cost, time committment, and training).

- Additional research is needed to develop validated and clinically applicable objective tools to assess vigilance, sleepiness, and fatigue.

DISCLOSURE

Dr I. Gurubhagavatula is principal investigator of an American Academy of Sleep Medicine Foundation Strategic Research Award.

FUNDING

AASM Foundation Award #192-SR-18.

REFERENCES

1. Kroenke K, Arrington ME, Mangelsdorff AD. The prevalence of symptoms in medical outpatients and the adequacy of therapy. Arch Intern Med 1990;150(8):1685–9.
2. Bates DW, Schmitt W, Buchwald D, et al. Prevalence of fatigue and chronic fatigue syndrome in a primary care practice. Arch Intern Med 1993; 153(24):2759–65.
3. Fuhrer R, Wessely S. The epidemiology of fatigue and depression: a French primary-care study. Psychol Med 1995;25(5):895–905.
4. Young TB. Epidemiology of daytime sleepiness: definitions, symptomatology, and prevalence. J Clin Psychiatry 2004;65(Suppl 16):12–6.
5. Gandhi KD, Mansukhani MP, Silber MH, et al. Excessive daytime sleepiness: a clinical review. Mayo Clin Proc 2021;96(5):1288–301 [published correction appears in Mayo Clin Proc. 2021 Oct; 96(10):2729].
6. Tefft BC. *The Prevalence and Impact of drowsy driving*(technical report). Washington, DC: AAA Foundation for Traffic Safety; 2010.
7. National Highway Traffic Safety Administration. Traffic safety facts: drowsy driving. Washington, DC: US Department of Transportation; 2011.
8. Bioulac S, Micoulaud-Franchi JA, Arnaud M, et al. Risk of motor vehicle accidents related to

sleepiness at the wheel: a systematic review and meta-analysis. Sleep 2017;40(10). https://doi.org/ 10.1093/sleep/zsx134 [Erratum in: Sleep. 2018 Jul 1;41(7)].
9. Gurubhagavatula I, Barger LK, Barnes CM, et al. Guiding principles for determining work shift duration and addressing the effects of work shift duration on performance, safety, and health: guidance from the American Academy of Sleep Medicine and the Sleep Research Society. Sleep 2021; 44(11):zsab161.
10. Chellappa SL, Morris CJ, Scheer FAJL. Daily circadian misalignment impairs human cognitive performance task-dependently. Sci Rep 2018;8(1):3041.
11. Folkard S, Lombardi DA. Modeling the impact of the components of long work hours on injuries and "accidents". Am J Ind Med 2006;49(11):953–63.
12. Institute of Medicine (US) Committee on Sleep Medicine and Research. In: Colten HR, Altevogt BM, editors. Sleep disorders and sleep deprivation: an unmet public health problem. Washington, DC: National Academies Press (US); 2006. 3, Extent and Health Consequences of Chronic Sleep Loss and Sleep Disorders. Available at: https://www.ncbi.nlm. nih.gov/books/NBK19961/.
13. Medic G, Wille M, Hemels ME. Short- and long-term health consequences of sleep disruption. Nat Sci Sleep 2017;9:151–61. PMID: 28579842; PMCID: PMC5449130.
14. Stone P, Richards M, Hardy J. Fatigue in patients with cancer. Eur J Cancer 1998;34(11):1670–6.
15. Kluger BM, Krupp LB, Enoka RM. Fatigue and fatigability in neurologic illnesses: proposal for a unified taxonomy. Neurology 2013;80(4):409–16.
16. Shen J, Barbera J, Shapiro CM. Distinguishing sleepiness and fatigue: focus on definition and measurement. Sleep Med Rev 2006;10(1):63–76.
17. van Schie MKM, Lammers GJ, Fronczek R, et al. Vigilance: discussion of related concepts and proposal for a definition. Sleep Med 2021;83:175–81.
18. BY Sunwoo, Jackson N, Maislin G, et al. Reliability of a single objective measure in assessing sleepiness. Sleep 2012;35(1):149–58.
19. Johns MW. A new method for measuring daytime sleepiness: the Epworth sleepiness scale. Sleep 1991;14(6):540–5.
20. Shprecher DR, Adler CH, Zhang N, et al. Do Parkinson disease subject and caregiver-reported Epworth sleepiness scale responses correlate? Clin Neurol Neurosurg 2020;192:105728.
21. Sap-Anan N, Pascoe M, Wang L, et al. The Epworth Sleepiness Scale in epilepsy: internal consistency and disease-related associations. Epilepsy Behav 2021;121(Pt A):108099.
22. Mills RJ, Koufali M, Sharma A, et al. Is the Epworth sleepiness scale suitable for use in stroke? Top Stroke Rehabil 2013;20(6):493–9.

23. Wang YG, Menno D, Chen A, et al. Validation of the Epworth Sleepiness Scale for Children and Adolescents (ESS-Chad) questionnaire in pediatric patients with narcolepsy with cataplexy aged 7-16 years. Sleep Med 2022;89:78–84.

24. Ahmed AE, Fatani A, Al-Harbi A, et al. Validation of the Arabic version of the Epworth sleepiness scale. J Epidemiol Glob Health 2014;4(4):297–302.

25. Chiner E, Arriero JM, Signes-Costa J, et al. Validación de la versión española del test de somnolencia Epworth en pacientes con síndrome de apnea de sueño [Validation of the Spanish version of the Epworth Sleepiness Scale in patients with a sleep apnea syndrome]. Arch Bronconeumol 1999;35(9):422–7.

26. Kaminska M, Jobin V, Mayer P, et al. The Epworth Sleepiness Scale: self-administration versus administration by the physician, and validation of a French version. Can Respir J 2010;17(2):e27–34.

27. Chen NH, Johns MW, Li HY, et al. Validation of a Chinese version of the Epworth sleepiness scale. Qual Life Res 2002;11(8):817–21.

28. Kanabar K, Sharma SK, Sreenivas V, et al. Validation of a Hindi version of the Epworth sleepiness scale (ESS) at AIIMS, New Delhi in sleep-disordered breathing. Sleep Breath 2016;20(4):1225–30.

29. Bertolazi AN, Fagondes SC, Hoff LS, et al. Portuguese-language version of the Epworth sleepiness scale: validation for use in Brazil. J Bras Pneumol 2009;35(9):877–83.

30. Grewe FA, Roeder M, Bradicich M, et al. Low repeatability of Epworth Sleepiness Scale after short intervals in a sleep clinic population. J Clin Sleep Med 2020;16(5):757–64.

31. Walker NA, Sunderram J, Zhang P, et al. Clinical utility of the Epworth sleepiness scale. Sleep Breath 2020;24(4):1759–65.

32. Herscovitch J, Broughton R. Sensitivity of the stanford sleepiness scale to the effects of cumulative partial sleep deprivation and recovery oversleeping. Sleep 1981;4(1):83–91.

33. Hoddes E, Dement W, Zarcone V. The history and use of the stanford sleepiness scale. Psychophysiology 1972;9:150.

34. Hoddes E, Zarcone V, Smythe H, et al. Quantification of sleepiness: a new approach. Psychophysiology 1973;10(4):431–6.

35. Mitler MM, Miller JC. Methods of testing for sleepiness [corrected]. Behav Med 1996;21(4):171–83 [Erratum in: Behav Med 1996 Spring;22(1):table of contents].

36. Dement WC, Carskadon MA, Richardson GS. Excessive daytime sleepiness in the sleep apnea syndrome. In: Guilleminault C, Dement WC, editors. Sleep apnea syndromes. New York: Alan R. Liss; 1978. p. 23–46.

37. Akerstedt T, Gillberg M. Subjective and objective sleepiness in the active individual. Int J Neurosci 1990;52(1–2):29–37.

38. Reyner LA, Horne JA. Falling asleep whilst driving: are drivers aware of prior sleepiness? Int J Legal Med 1998;111:120–3.

39. Horne JA, Baulk SD. Awareness of sleepiness when driving. Psychophysiology 2004;41:161–5.

40. Kaida K, Takahashi M, Akerstedt T, et al. Validation of the Karolinska sleepiness scale against performance and EEG variables. Clin Neurophysiol 2006;117(7):1574–81.

41. Axelsson J, Åkerstedt T, Kecklund G, et al. Tolerance to shift work-how does it relate to sleep and wakefulness? Int Arch Occup Environ Health 2004;77:121–9.

42. Gillberg M. Subjective alertness and sleep quality in connection with permanent 12-hour day and night shifts. Scand J Work Environ Health 1998;24(Suppl. 3).76–80.

43. Härmä M, Sallinen M, Ranta R, et al. The effect of an irregular shift system on sleepiness at work in train drivers and railway traffic controllers. J Sleep Res 2002;11:141–51.

44. Ingre M, Kecklund G, Åkerstedt T, et al. Variation in sleepiness during early morning shifts: a mixed model approach to an experimental field study of train drivers. Chronobiol Int 2004;21:973–90.

45. Sallinen M, Härmä M, Akila R, et al. The effects of sleep debt and monotonous work on sleepiness and performance during a 12-h dayshift. J Sleep Res 2004;13:285–94.

46. Suhner A, Schlagenhauf P, Johnson R, et al. Comparative study to determine the optimal melatonin dosage form for the alleviation of jet lag. Chronobiol Int 1998;15:655–66.

47. Mary A. Carskadon, guidelines for the multiple sleep latency test (MSLT): a standard measure of sleepiness. Sleep 1986;9(4):519–24.

48. Carskadon MA, Dement WC. Effects of total sleep loss on sleep tendency. Percept Mot Skills 1979;48(2):495–506.

49. Gurubhagavatula I. Consequences of obstructive sleep apnoea. Indian J Med Res 2010;131:188–95.

50. Krahn LE, Arand DL, Avidan AY, et al. Recommended protocols for the multiple sleep latency test and maintenance of wakefulness test in adults: guidance from the American Academy of sleep medicine [published correction appears in J Clin sleep med. 2022 Aug 1;18(8):2089]. J Clin Sleep Med 2021;17(12):2489–98.

51. Goldbart A, Peppard P, Finn L, et al. Narcolepsy and predictors of positive MSLTs in the Wisconsin sleep cohort. Sleep 2014;37(6):1043–51.

52. Cairns A, Trotti LM, Bogan R. Demographic and nap-related variance of the MSLT: results from 2,498 suspected hypersomnia patients: clinical MSLT variance. Sleep Med 2019;55:115–23.

53. Bonnet MH, Arand DL. Sleepiness as measured by modified multiple sleep latency testing varies as a function of preceding activity. Sleep 1998;21(5):477–83.

54. Bonnet MH, Arand DL. 24-Hour metabolic rate in insomniacs and matched normal sleepers. Sleep 1995;18(7):581–8.

55. Stepanski E, Zorick F, Roehrs T, et al. Daytime alertness in patients with chronic insomnia compared with asymptomatic control subjects. Sleep 1988;11(1):54–60.

56. Schneider-Helmert D. Twenty-four-hour sleep-wake function and personality patterns in chronic insomniacs and healthy controls. Sleep 1987;10(5):452–62.

57. Stepanski E, Zorick F, Roehrs T, et al. Effects of sleep deprivation on daytime sleepiness in primary insomnia. Sleep 2000;23(2):215–9.

58. Muza R, Lykouras D, Rees K. The utility of a 5(th) nap in multiple sleep latency test. J Thorac Dis 2016;8(2):282–6.

59. Doghramji K, Mitler MM, Sangal RB, et al. A normative study of the maintenance of wakefulness test (MWT). Electroencephalogr Clin Neurophysiol 1997;103(5):554–62.

60. Banks S, Barnes M, Tarquinio N, et al. The maintenance of wakefulness test in normal healthy subjects. Sleep 2004;27(4):799–802.

61. Anniss AM, Young A, O'Driscoll DM. Microsleep assessment enhances interpretation of the maintenance of wakefulness test. J Clin Sleep Med 2021;17(8):1571–8.

62. Philip P, Guichard K, Strauss M, et al. Maintenance of wakefulness test: how does it predict accident risk in patients with sleep disorders? Sleep Med 2021;77:249–55.

63. Bennett LS, Stradling JR, Davies RJ. A behavioural test to assess daytime sleepiness in obstructive sleep apnoea. J Sleep Res 1997;6(2):142–5.

64. Priest B, Brichard C, Aubert G, et al. Microsleep during a simplified maintenance of wakefulness test. A validation study of the OSLER test. Am J Respir Crit Care Med 2001;163(7):1619–25.

65. Larrateguy LD, Pais CM, Larrateguy LI, et al. Simplified sleep resistance test for daytime sleepiness detection. Sleep Sci 2021;14(2):164–8.

66. LOWENSTEIN O, LOEWENFELD IE. Influence of retinal adaptation upon the pupillary reflex to light in normal man. Part I. Effect of adaptation to bright light on the pupillary threshold. Am J Ophthalmol 1959;48(5):536–50. Pt 2.

67. Yoss RE, Moyer NJ, Ogle KN. The pupillogram and narcolepsy. A method to measure decreased levels of wakefulness. Neurology 1969;19(10):921–8.

68. Yoss RE, Moyer NJ, Hollenhorst RW. Pupil size and spontaneous pupillary waves associated with alertness, drowsiness, and sleep. Neurology 1970;20(6):545–54.

69. McLaren JW, Hauri PJ, Lin SC, et al. Pupillometry in clinically sleepy patients. Sleep Med 2002;3(4):347–52.

70. Dinges DF, Grace R. PERCLOS: A valid psychophysiological measure of alertness as assessed by psychomotor vigilance. Federal Highway Administration, Publication no. FHWA-MCRT-98-006. Washington, DC: US Department of Transportation; 1998.

71. Manousakis JE, Maccora J, Anderson C. The validity of the pupillographic sleepiness test at shorter task durations. Behav Res Methods 2021;53(4):1488–501.

72. Shi L, Zheng L, Jin D, et al. Assessment of Combination of automated pupillometry and heart rate variability to detect driving fatigue. Front Public Health 2022;10:828428.

73. Bastuji H, García-Larrea L. Evoked potentials as a tool for the investigation of human sleep. Sleep Med Rev 1999;3(1):23–45.

74. Alloway CE, Ogilvie RD, Shapiro CM. The alpha attenuation test: assessing excessive daytime sleepiness in narcolepsy-cataplexy. Sleep 1997;20(4):258–66.

75. Putilov AA, Donskaya OG. Alpha attenuation soon after closing the eyes as an objective indicator of sleepiness. Clin Exp Pharmacol Physiol 2014;41(12):956–64.

76. Krupp LB, LaRocca NG, Muir-Nash J, et al. The fatigue severity scale. Application to patients with multiple sclerosis and systemic lupus erythematosus. Arch Neurol 1989;46(10):1121–3.

77. Chalder T, Berelowitz G, Pawlikowska T, et al. Development of a fatigue scale. J Psychosom Res 1993;37(2):147–53.

78. Dittner AJ, Wessely SC, Brown RG. The assessment of fatigue: a practical guide for clinicians and researchers. J Psychosom Res 2004;56(2):157–70.

79. Fisk JD, Ritvo PG, Ross L, et al. Measuring the functional impact of fatigue: initial validation of the fatigue impact scale. Clin Infect Dis 1994;18(Suppl 1):S79–83.

80. Lopes J, AraÚjo HAGO, Smaili SM. Fatigue in Parkinson's disease: Brazilian validation of the modified fatigue impact scale. Arq Neuropsiquiatr 2020;78(8):473–80.

81. Frith J, Newton J. Fatigue impact scale. Occup Med (Lond) 2010;60(2):159.

82. Ritvo P, Fischer J, Miller D, et al. Multiple sclerosis quality of life inventory: a user's manual. New York: National Multiple Sclerosis Society; 1997. p. 65.

83. Larson RD. Psychometric properties of the modified fatigue impact scale. Int J MS Care 2013;15(1):15–20.

84. Mensen JM, Dang JS, Stets AJ, et al. The effects of real-time performance feedback and performance emphasis on the sustained attention to response task (SART). Psychol Res 2022;86(6):1972–9.

85. Dinges DF, Powell JW. Microcomputer analyses of performance on a portable, simple visual RT task during sustained operations. Behav Res Methods Instrum Comput 1985;17:652–5.

86. Basner M, Hermosillo E, Nasrini J, et al. Repeated administration effects on psychomotor vigilance test performance. Sleep 2018;41(1). https://doi.org/10.1093/sleep/zsx187.

87. Antler CA, Yamazaki EM, Casale CE, et al. The 3-minute psychomotor vigilance test demonstrates inadequate Convergent validity relative to the 10-minute psychomotor vigilance test across sleep loss and recovery. Front Neurosci 2022;16:815697.

88. George CF, Boudreau AC, Smiley A. Comparison of simulated driving performance in narcolepsy and sleep apnea patients. Sleep 1996;19(9):711–7.

89. Robertson IH, Manly T, Andrade J, et al. 'Oops!': performance correlates of everyday attentional failures in traumatic brain injured and normal subjects. Neuropsychologia 1997;35(6):747–58.

90. Rizzo R, Knight SP, Davis JRC, et al. Longitudinal study on sustained attention to response task (SART): Clustering approach for mobility and cognitive decline. Geriatrics 2022;7(3):51.

91. Whyte J, Grieb-Neff P, Gantz C, et al. Measuring sustained attention after traumatic brain injury: differences in key findings from the sustained attention to response task (SART). Neuropsychologia 2006;44(10):2007–14.

92. Head J, Tenan MS, Tweedell AJ, et al. Prior mental fatigue Impairs marksmanship decision performance. Front Physiol 2017;8:680.

93. Munnik A, Näswall K, Woodward G, et al. The quick and the dead: a paradigm for studying friendly fire. Appl Ergon 2020;84:103032.

94. American Academy of Sleep Medicine Board of Directors, Watson NF, Morgenthaler T, Chervin R, et al. Confronting drowsy driving: the American Academy of sleep medicine perspective. J Clin Sleep Med 2015;11(11):1335–6.

95. Maia Q, Grandner MA, Findley J, et al. Short and long sleep duration and risk of drowsy driving and the role of subjective sleep insufficiency. Accid Anal Prev 2013;59:618–22.

96. Gurubhagavatula I, Sullivan SS. Screening for sleepiness and sleep disorders in commercial drivers. Sleep Med Clin 2019;14(4):453–62.

97. Weaver MD, Vetter C, Rajaratnam SMW, et al. Sleep disorders, depression and anxiety are associated with adverse safety outcomes in healthcare workers: a prospective cohort study. J Sleep Res 2018;27(6):e12722.

98. Kancherla BS, Upender R, Collen JF, et al. What is the role of sleep in physician burnout? J Clin Sleep Med 2020;16(5):807–10.

99. Kancherla BS, Upender R, Collen JF, et al. Sleep, fatigue and burnout among physicians: an American Academy of Sleep Medicine position statement. J Clin Sleep Med 2020;16(5):803–5.

100. Weaver MD, Robbins R, Quan SF, et al. Association of sleep disorders with physician burnout. JAMA Netw Open. 2020;3(10):e2023256.

101. Shea JA, Bellini LM, Dinges DF, et al. Impact of protected sleep period for internal medicine interns on overnight call on depression, burnout, and empathy. J Grad Med Educ 2014;6(2):256–63.

102. Sørengaard TA, Saksvik-Lehouillier I. Associations between burnout symptoms and sleep among workers during the COVID-19 pandemic. Sleep Med 2022;90:199–203.

103. Klösch G, Zeitlhofer J, Ipsiroglu O. Revisiting the concept of vigilance. Front Psychiatry 2022;13:874757.

Dawn of a New Dawn
Advances in Sleep Health to Optimize Performance

Alice D. LaGoy, PhD[a,b,1], Andrew G. Kubala, PhD[a,b,1], Sean Deering, BS[a,b], Anne Germain, PhD[c,2], Rachel R. Markwald, PhD[a,*]

KEYWORDS

- Military • High-risk occupations • Wearables • Fatigue risk • Sleep interventions

KEY POINTS

- Sleep health is critical to performance and further investigation is warranted to explore how sleep characteristics such as sleep regularity or timing are directly related to performance across high-risk populations (eg, military, health care workers, firefighters).
- Many wearable health monitors and research grade actigraphs can estimate sleep time in overnight sleep contexts and with further investigation, may be accessible support tools for sleep health monitoring and improvement strategies.
- Advances in technologies and approaches to mitigate poor sleep health such as non-invasive brain stimulation, timed caffeine or light administration, and remote behavioral health interventions could prove to alleviate performance decrements. However, these strategies need to be further studied in ecological models with performance-oriented outcomes and risk assessment.

SLEEP HEALTH AND PERFORMANCE

Sleep is a multifaceted process that cycles through different stages and is regulated by homeostatic and circadian influences. Sleep stages are defined by electroencephalography (EEG) assessed patterns in brain wave activity and are categorized into rapid eye movement (REM) and non-REM (NREM) sleep, the latter of which is further divided into NREM stages N1, N2, and N3.[1] These stages may serve different functions. For example, N3 (slow wave sleep [SWS]) may contribute to the restorative function of sleep[2]

while REM may contribute more to emotional memory processing.[3] Within the past decade, the sleep field has expanded beyond focusing on sleep duration and stages, to further operationalize sleep health as a multidimensional construct including other sleep characteristics such as the timing, regularity, continuity, and overall subjective satisfaction of sleep.[4,5] This broader focus has led to initiatives and advances across the sleep field to understand relationships between multiple sleep characteristics and health risk.[6] Regarding physical and cognitive performance, particularly in high performing groups such as the military or

---

Author Note: The author is a military service member or employee of the U.S. Government. This work was prepared as part of my official duties. Title 17, U.S.C §105 provides that copyright protection under this title is not available for any work of the U.S. Government. Title 17, U.S.C §101 defines a U.S. Government work as work prepared by a military service member or employee of the U.S. Government as part of that person's official duties. The views expressed in this article are those of the authors and do not necessarily reflect the official policy or position of the Department of the Navy, Department of Defense, nor the U.S. Government.

[a] Sleep, Tactical Efficiency, and Endurance Laboratory, Warfighter Performance Department, Naval Health Research Center, 140 Sylvester Road, San Diego, CA 92106, USA; [b] Leidos, Inc., San Diego, CA, USA; [c] NOCTEM Health Inc., Pittsburgh, PA, USA

[1] Co-first authors.

[2] Present address: 218 Oakland Avenue, Pittsburgh PA 15213.

* Corresponding author.

E-mail address: rachel.r.markwald.civ@health.mil

athletics, much of the literature still focuses on sleep duration[7,8] as the primary outcome of interest.

Sleep duration plays a critical role in performance through effects on cognitive, physical, and skilled function. These relationships are illustrated by the consistent and substantial deficits in cognitive performance (ie, attention, working memory, cognitive flexibility, response inhibition, and decision-making) that follow extended wakefulness.[9,10] Deficits in physical and skilled (eg, marksmanship, coordination, athletic) performance are also observed following sleep loss.[8,11,12] Without sleep, cognitive and physical recovery may also be compromised. Sleep, but not quiet restfulness, restored cognitive function following extended wakefulness and contributed to muscle recovery following physical exertion.[13,14] Such effects may be related to slow wave activity (SWA; 0.5–4 Hz activity), which characterizes SWS and may promote conditions favorable for cognitive and physical recovery.[2,14]

Although less examined, other sleep characteristics such as regularity, fragmentation, and timing may also impact performance.[15-17] In 2 select studies, higher sleep regularity (ie, more consistent onset and offset of sleep) predicted better academic performance in undergraduate students,[18,19] while participants with more consistent sleep schedules during a 13 month stay in Antarctica were protected against deficits in psychomotor function compared with participants with more variable sleep timing.[20] More investigation is needed regarding the combined effects of multiple sleep characteristics on performance across various populations.

Despite the importance of sleep for optimal performance, high-performing populations such as athletes and operational personnel are often subjected to demands that challenge the maintenance of regular, sufficient, consolidated, and restorative sleep.[21-26] Suboptimal sleep in these populations contributes to worse performance (eg, basketball game or combat drill performance) and increased injury risk.[17,27-29] Early morning training and/or competitions, pre-competition anxiety, and frequent travel contribute to poor sleep in athletes,[22,24] while operational schedules (eg, nightshift work, rotating/extended shifts, unpredictable work hours) and poor sleeping environments contribute to poor sleep in operational populations (eg, military personnel, medical professionals, firefighters).[25,30] Ecological and easily accessible sleep monitoring methods may allow for early identification of disrupted sleep and early intervention to improve sleep, prior to observable deficits in performance. Also important is identifying strategies to optimize sleep and to mitigate sleep loss-related risk. However, the aforementioned barriers to sleep may not only impact sleep health (thereby compromising performance) but may also affect the implementation of sleep health interventions. In the following sections, we will outline select sleep health advances and will detail the implementation potential of these advances in real-world settings.

ADVANCES IN SLEEP HEALTH MONITORING TO OPTIMIZE PERFORMANCE
Wearables

Wearables (ie, commercially available sleep and physiological tracking devices) are widely used, relatively inexpensive and readily available. The ability to utilize wearables to perform real-time, prospective sleep monitoring and targeted real-world interventions to improve sleep and optimize performance could potentially benefit individuals with suboptimal sleep patterns, including athletes and operational groups. For such interventions to be successful, it must first be possible to accurately measure sleep in real-world settings. A number of research studies have directly compared sleep measurements obtained from wearables to research-grade actigraphy and the gold standard sleep measurement technique, polysomnography (PSG), which are significantly costlier and less accessible in non-clinical settings. These studies found that certain wearables (eg, Fitbit, Fatigue Science ReadiBand, Oura ring) could accurately obtain key sleep/wake metrics, with some performing as well or better than actigraphy relative to PSG or mobile EEG.[31-34]

Furthermore, studies that have used actigraphy and wearables to monitor sleep and provide individually tailored feedback have shown that it is possible to improve sleep health in this manner.[35,36] Of note, Adler and colleagues found that combining actigraphy with personalized sleep reports increased sleep duration and self-reported sleep quality in Army soldiers.[35] Additionally, wearable data can be fed into computational models and aggregated with other data sources to provide meaningful insights related to sleep and activity levels, which in turn can potentially be used to optimize sleep and performance.[37,38]

Biomathematical Models and Fatigue Risk Management Systems

Biomathematical models of fatigue predict alertness based on work schedules, sleep-wake schedules and/or objective sleep data.[39] Parameters included in the models capture homeostatic sleep pressure, which increases with time awake, circadian-mediated alertness changes, which vary across time-of-day, and sleep inertia (ie, the grogginess that occurs upon awakening).[40,41] Additional models (described below) also consider the effects of caffeine intake.[42] By incorporating these models into fatigue risk management systems, heightened fatigue risk can be predicted and mitigated before resulting in compromised performance.[43] Aviation and trucking industries have used fatigue risk management systems to inform scheduling practices and fatigue mitigation strategy use, which maintains overall performance and individual safety.[43] Continued refinement of these models has allowed them to be generalizable across self-report and objective measures and across different operational populations (ie, policeman and truck drivers).[39,40]

Several advances in technology may increase future use of biomathematical models and fatigue risk management systems. Within real-world settings, objective sleep–wake data have traditionally been difficult to collect, but the recent advancements in wearable technology may reduce this difficulty, allowing for further improvement of models.[38,44] Further, as stated above, data from these wearable devices can be integrated with biomathematical models and presented in mobile and web-based applications to provide actionable, interpretable, and real-time information regarding fatigue risk. Still, while biomathematical models effectively predict alertness, their ability to predict other aspects of real-world performance remains unknown. Further, optimization of biomathematical models with objective data requires access to raw data for effective algorithm development, which is often not readily available from commercial wearables. Such access is needed for broad validation, implementation, and evaluation of models.

ADVANCES IN SLEEP HEALTH INTERVENTIONS TO OPTIMIZE AND MAINTAIN PERFORMANCE
Sleep Education and Behavior

Sleep health education and behavioral interventions may be readily implemented and tailored to the specific needs of different populations. Such programs often provide information regarding sleep timing, functional implications of sleep, caffeine use, and light exposure. Sleep education programs have largely resulted in positive changes in sleep behaviors (eg, longer duration, better quality, improved timing).[45–52] However, whether these changes in sleep are long-lasting or improve performance remains less clear. In a sample of 24 rugby league athletes, 2 weeks of sleep health education effectively altered sleep behaviors (ie, timing and duration), but these changes were not maintained

a month after the program.[45] Of note, associations between sleep and performance were not examined. These findings illustrate the difficulty of making long-lasting behavioral changes. Combining sleep health education programs with continuous sleep monitoring and real-time feedback (described above) may increase the likelihood of persistent behavioral changes.

Further, inconsistency surrounds the potential effects of sleep health interventions on performance. Some studies have reported no effects of sleep health education on performance outcomes,[46,48,49] while others have reported benefits to aspects of physical performance (ie, sprint time and countermovement jumps) when combined with bright light exposure.[47] While sleep health education may be an important component of sleep health interventions, the long-term and performance-related implications of this education must be further established. Relatedly, the effectiveness of combining sleep health education with additional interventions, such as continuous objective monitoring,[35] to enhance performance must be further explored.

Sleep Banking, Napping, and Sleep Extension

The benefits of obtaining more sleep and napping prior to important events or periods of restricted sleep have long been described[53–55] and have been further supported in recent work. The practice of sleep extension involves increasing the time-in-bed opportunity for sleep, allowing for maximal sleep to occur.[56] The benefits of sleep extension are diverse, affecting both cognitive and physical performance.[57–59] Following four nights of sleep extension resulting in ~1.4 more hours of sleep by Reserve Officers' Training Corps cadets, reaction time, executive function, motivation, and broad jump performance improved.[58] Further, multiple weeks of sleep extension in well-trained athletes led to improved skilled performance (ie, basketball shooting and tennis serve accuracy), thereby demonstrating benefits of sleep extension on real-world performance within naturalistic settings.[60,61] Sleep extension when used to achieve more sleep than usual to prepare for sleep loss is termed sleep banking, a practice that may offset/protect against sleep loss-related performance decrements.[56,62,63]

Naps may similarly be used to "bank sleep" before sleep loss to attenuate sleep loss-related deficits.[64] Napping can also benefit cognitive and physical performance in well-rested individuals.[65] Recent work has detailed beneficial effects of various nap durations (40–90 min) on repeated sprint performance and on perceptual and physiological responses to physical exertion.[66–69] Still, the implementation of napping as a fatigue mitigation and performance optimization strategy in operational settings remains controversial.[70] Sleep inertia may be more severe following naps during extended wakefulness or during night-shifts.[71] For individuals working on-call shifts and/or nightshifts, sleep inertia may compromise job performance immediately upon awakening. Combining naps with other sleep heath interventions such as caffeine[72] and light exposure[73,74] (described below) may mitigate sleep inertia and augment the beneficial effects of naps on performance, but further work is needed to better understand these interactive effects.

Napping, sleep extension, and sleep banking have been effectively implemented across athletic and operational populations, but these strategies may not address all barriers to sleep experienced by high-performers (eg, poor sleeping environments, variable sleep schedules, work-related time constraints). Therefore, increasing sleep duration through naps or sleep extension may not always be effective or even possible within real-world settings.

Caffeine

The use of caffeine to increase alertness and mitigate detrimental effects of sleep loss (to an extent) has been well described.[75–81] It must be noted that as sleep loss becomes more severe (eg, after 5 nights with 4 hours of sleep), caffeine may no longer prevent alertness decrements.[81] Still, a recent position statement from the International Society of Sports Nutrition outlined the benefits of caffeine on physical and cognitive performance, and provided recommendations for use.[82] The magnitude of these benefits varies based on individual sensitivity to caffeine, and the dose and timing of caffeine intake. Intake within 6 hours of bedtime may compromise sleep, while excessive single or combined doses of caffeine may additionally compromise performance and recovery following sleep loss.[81] Therefore, proper caffeine dosing (0.5–6 mg/kg body weight depending on the purpose) and timing are essential to maximizing the potential benefits of caffeine.[77,82] To this end, the 2B-Alert mobile application was developed to provide recommendations for caffeine dosing to minimize neurobehavioral impairment.[42] Feedback provided by 2B-Alert may better allow individuals to maintain neurobehavioral function during sleep loss. Still, additional work is needed to optimize the models used by 2B-Alert to reflect individual responses to sleep loss and caffeine use relative to the next sleep opportunity.[83]

When used proactively, caffeine may also mitigate detrimental effects of sleep inertia on alertness and performance following a nap.[72,84,85] Caffeine intake before an afternoon nap increased alertness (both subjective and neurobehavioral responses) following the nap, without disrupting sleep during the nap. Further, Romdhani and colleagues suggested that combining a nap with caffeine intake improved repeated sprint performance greater than either alone.

Overall, caffeine may effectively mitigate sleep loss- and sleep inertia-related performance decrements, but additional work is needed to better predict individual responses to caffeine and to examine sleep inertia mitigation in larger samples.

Light Interventions

Exposure to bright (>900 lux), blue (~480 nm), or red (~630 nm) light impacts sleep–wake rhythms, increases alertness and improves mood, cognitive, and physical performance. Through projections from specialized, light-sensitive retinal cells to the suprachiasmatic nucleus (SCN; circadian pacemaker), light exerts a strong influence on circadian rhythms.[86] Relatedly, effects of light on sleep depend on time-of-day; more light throughout the day may benefit sleep, while light immediately before sleep results in delayed and disrupted sleep.[87] These disruptive effects may be less pronounced following red light exposure.[88] Blocking or minimizing blue light exposure prior to bed may therefore promote optimal sleep health.[89] The specialized retinal cells also project to subcortical regions related to alertness and cortical regions related to cognitive function.[86] Accordingly, prolonged/consistent light exposure, achieved through replacement of light bulbs emitting different light spectra, mitigated alertness decrements throughout nightshift work.[90] Further, shorter duration exposures to light, achieved through light boxes or specialized eyewear, have also resulted in benefits to cognitive and physical performance. Bright, blue, and red light interventions may effectively mitigate jet lag,[47,91,92] sleep inertia,[71,73,74,93,94] the early afternoon dip in alertness/performance,[93,95] and disruptions related to nightshift work.[90]

The ability of light interventions to mitigate sleep inertia severity and to increase alertness may be of particular importance to operational populations, who may need to execute safety-critical work demands shortly after awakening. One hour of exposure to polychromatic light after being awoken from SWS (which may increase sleep inertia severity) reduced sleepiness and improved mood and neurobehavioral performance, highlighting the potential of bright light to serve as a reactive countermeasure to sleep inertia.[74] Similar effects of bright light have been found following an afternoon nap, with benefits on mood, alertness, and cognitive flexibility described.[95]

Beneficial effects of light have been observed across different use-cases, doses, and administration techniques, which demonstrates the potential for broader implementation of light interventions across different field settings. Still, the minimum dose (eg, light intensity and exposure duration) to elicit beneficial and prolonged effects has not been established. Such knowledge would inform the implementation potential of light interventions within operational settings.

Non-invasive Brain Stimulation

Non-invasive brain stimulation (NIBS), including transcranial magnetic (TMS), transcranial electric (TES), and auditory stimulation may also enhance sleep and optimize performance.[96] TMS and TES involve applying magnetic and electric pulses, respectively, to the scalp, which modulates the excitability of underlying brain regions allowing for targeted manipulation of function. When applied during wakefulness, TMS and TES can improve cognitive and sensorimotor performance, including attention, memory, logical reasoning, perceptual capabilities, and motor function.[97] Relatedly, TMS and TES may protect against cognitive deficits during sleep loss.[98–101] For example, TES maintained attention and working memory during 30+ hours of wakefulness.[100,101] TMS and TES may also optimize performance through sleep enhancement by increasing SWA. Application of TMS and TES during wakefulness results in use-dependent (ie, stimulation-site specific) increases in SWA during the subsequent sleep bout.[102] Similarly, low-frequency (~0.75 Hz) TMS and TES can be applied during sleep to directly induce slow waves and entrain site-specific brain activity to the stimulation frequency.[102–108] TES-mediated SWA enhancement has been associated with improved cognitive function,[107,109,110] consistent with known associations between use-dependent SWA modulation and performance.[96,111–113] Conversely, functional benefits of TMS-mediated SWA changes have yet to be quantified, which may be due to the increased difficulty of administering TMS during sleep relative to other NIBS modalities—a factor that may also limit its implementation in the field.

Auditory stimulation applied during sleep can also enhance SWA and improve performance.

Auditory stimulation takes advantage of naturally occurring brain responses to sensory input during sleep to induce and entrain brain activity. During closed-loop protocols, auditory tones are played during the up-state of naturally occurring slow waves to increase local neuronal synchrony, thereby augmenting ongoing slow waves and increasing SWA throughout the night.[114–119] Similar to TES, potential benefits to verbal fluency, declarative memory, and working memory are found following auditory stimulation,[96,111,119] but given the modest effect sizes observed, additional work is needed to characterize the functional significance of performance changes.

NIBS techniques have gained notoriety for their ability to increase SWA, thereby potentially increasing the restorative nature of sleep. For individuals experiencing poor sleep in operational or high-tempo environments, the ability to enhance the functional benefits of sleep could have substantial implications on well-being, performance, and safety. Still, before NIBS can/should be recommended for use in real-world settings, we must further quantify the functional meaningfulness of performance benefits, the ability to effect change in real-world performance within field settings, and the acute versus chronic effects of stimulation on health and performance.[120]

DISCUSSION

Advances in strategies to monitor and improve sleep health provide opportunities to optimize performance through sleep (**Fig. 1**). Protecting and/or improving sleep health can benefit health, well-being, performance, and recovery. Of further importance, sleep health interventions may also attenuate sleep loss and sleep inertia-related deficits in function. The ability to protect alertness and performance, at least acutely, during periods of sleep loss may have substantial implications for operational populations who must maintain performance despite regular exposure to sleep loss. For example, military personnel may have limited ability to obtain sufficient sleep when conducting multi-day operations, an ability to maintain function or minimize performance deficits during these missions may increase the likelihood of mission success and minimize risk to military personnel.

Still, additional work is needed to address several critical gaps. First, as sleep is further examined from a multidimensional perspective, additional insights regarding the functional implications of sleep may be better understood. Second, the impact of sleep health interventions on

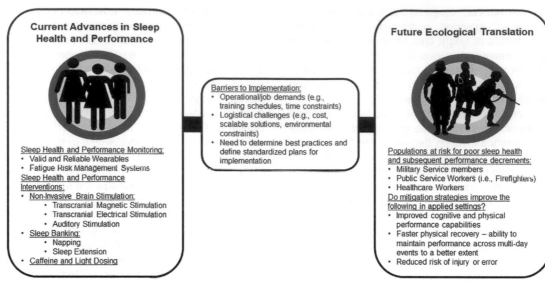

Fig. 1. Transitioning current advances in sleep health to at-risk populations.

real-world performance need to be further quantified across functionally relevant domains. Most studies examining sleep health monitoring or intervention strategies have been performed in laboratory settings and/or have quantified performance using standardized/controlled tasks that assess targeted aspects of performance (eg, attention, working memory). Although quantifying real-world performance can be challenging due to the dynamic and complex nature of these tasks, doing so is essential to understand the real-world implications of insufficient sleep. Third, further tailoring of the aforementioned advances is needed to increase the feasibility of implementing these advances in specific use-cases with different barriers to optimal sleep and different performance-related goals. Such barriers and goals may impact implementation feasibility and should therefore inform implementation strategies. By addressing these gaps, standardized practices and improved fatigue risk management systems may be developed to better identify, predict, and mitigate sleep loss-related impairments in real-world settings.

SUMMARY

In summary, optimal sleep health is essential for optimal performance but is often difficult to sustain for high-performing populations. Although there is substantial evidence detailing links between sleep and performance, and the efficacy of different sleep health interventions to improve sleep, additional work is needed to understand implications on performance in real-world settings. Further,

additional work is needed to increase the feasibility of implementations within real-world settings.

FUNDING

Work was supported by the Office of Naval Research under work unit no. N1701 and by the Military Operational Medicine Research Program/ Joint Program Committee 5 under work unit no. N2010.

CLINICS CARE POINTS

- Recent advances in commercially available sleep tracking devices have allowed for enhanced sleep monitoring capabilities, that, when combined with advances in biomathematical modeling may inform targeted performance optimization strategies.

- When sufficient sleep cannot be obtained, evidence-based use of sleep banking, caffeine, and light may attenuate performance deficits over an acute period.

- When considering implementation of sleep health interventions in real-world settings, barriers to implementation specific to the population of interest must be considered.

REFERENCES

1. Berry RB, Albertario CL, Harding SM, et al. The AASM manual for the scoring of sleep and associated events: rules, terminology and technical

specifications. Darien, IL: American Academy of Sleep Medicine; 2018.

2. Tononi G, Cirelli C. Sleep function and synaptic homeostasis. Sleep Med Rev 2006;10(1):49–62.

3. Genzel L, Spoormaker VI, Konrad BN, et al. The role of rapid eye movement sleep for amygdala-related memory processing. Neurobiol Learn Mem 2015;122:110–21.

4. Buysse DJ. Sleep health: can we define it? Does it matter? Sleep 2014;37(1):9–17.

5. Wallace ML, Yu L, Buysse DJ, et al. Multidimensional sleep health domains in older men and women: an actigraphy factor analysis. Sleep 2021;44(2):zsaa181.

6. Bowman MA, Kline CE, Buysse DJ, et al. Longitudinal association between depressive symptoms and multidimensional sleep health: the SWAN sleep study. Ann Behav Med 2021;55(7):641–52.

7. Watson AM. Sleep and Athletic Performance. Curr Sports Med Rep 2017;16(6):413–8.

8. Grandou C, Wallace L, Fullagar HHK, et al. The Effects of Sleep Loss on Military Physical Performance. Sports Med 2019;49(8):1159–72.

9. Pilcher JJ, Huffcutt AI. Effects of sleep deprivation on performance: a meta-analysis. Sleep 1996; 19(4):318–26.

10. Feld GB, Diekelmann S. Sleep smart—optimizing sleep for declarative learning and memory. Front Psychol 2015;6(622). https://doi.org/10.3389/fpsyg.2015.00622.

11. Fullagar HH, Skorski S, Duffield R, et al. Sleep and athletic performance: the effects of sleep loss on exercise performance, and physiological and cognitive responses to exercise. Sports Med 2015;45(2):161–86.

12. Charest J, Grandner MA. Sleep and Athletic Performance: Impacts on Physical Performance, Mental Performance, Injury Risk and Recovery, and Mental Health: An Update. Sleep Med Clin 2022;17(2): 263–82.

13. Mednick SC, Nakayama K, Cantero JL, et al. The restorative effect of naps on perceptual deterioration. Nat Neurosci 2002;5(7):677–81.

14. Chennaoui M, Vanneau T, Trignol A, et al. How does sleep help recovery from exercise-induced muscle injuries? J Sci Med Sport 2021;24(10):982–7.

15. Koa TB, Lo JC. Neurobehavioural functions during variable and stable short sleep schedules. J Sleep Res 2021;30(4):e13252.

16. Sletten TL, Sullivan JP, Arendt J, et al. The role of circadian phase in sleep and performance during Antarctic winter expeditions. J Pineal Res 2022; 73(2):e12817.

17. Jones JJ, Kirschen GW, Kancharla S, et al. Association between late-night tweeting and next-day game performance among professional basketball players. Sleep Health 2019;5(1):68–71.

18. Phillips AJK, Clerx WM, O'Brien CS, et al. Irregular sleep/wake patterns are associated with poorer academic performance and delayed circadian and sleep/wake timing. Sci Rep 2017;7(1):3216.

19. Bono TJ, Hill PL. Sleep quantity and variability during the first semester at university: implications for well-being and academic performance. Psychol Health Med 2022;27(4):931–6.

20. Mairesse O, MacDonald-Nethercott E, Neu D, et al. Preparing for Mars: human sleep and performance during a 13 month stay in Antarctica. Sleep 2018; 42(1).

21. Fox JL, Scanlan AT, Stanton R, et al. Losing Sleep Over It: Sleep in Basketball Players Affected by Game But Not Training Workloads. Int J Sports Physiol Perform 2020;15(8):1117–24.

22. Halson SL, Johnston RD, Appaneal RN, et al. Sleep Quality in Elite Athletes: Normative Values, Reliability and Understanding Contributors to Poor Sleep. Sports Med 2022;52(2):417–26.

23. Lastella M, Roach GD, Halson SL, et al. Sleep/wake behaviours of elite athletes from individual and team sports. Eur J Sport Sci 2015;15(2): 94–100.

24. Sargent C, Halson S, Roach GD. Sleep or swim? Early-morning training severely restricts the amount of sleep obtained by elite swimmers. Eur J Sport Sci 2014;14(Suppl 1):S310–5.

25. Good CH, Brager AJ, Capaldi VF, et al. Sleep in the United States Military. Neuropsychopharmacology 2020;45(1):176–91.

26. Seelig AD, Jacobson IG, Smith B, et al. Sleep Patterns Before, During, and After Deployment to Iraq and Afghanistan. Sleep 2010;33(12):1615–22.

27. Cook JD, Charest J, Walch O, et al. Associations of circadian change, travel distance, and their interaction with basketball performance: a retrospective analysis of 2014-2018 National Basketball Association data. Chronobiol Int 2022;39(10):1399–410.

28. Mantua J, Shevchik JD, Chaudhury S, et al. Sleep and Infantry Battle Drill Performance in Special Operations Soldiers. Aerosp Med Hum Perform 2022; 93(7):557–61.

29. Ritland BM, Naylor JA, Bessey AF, et al. Association between Self-Reported sleep Quality and Musculoskeletal Injury in Male Army Rangers. Military Medicine; 2021. p. usab488.

30. Patterson PD, Weaver MD, Hostler D, et al. The shift length, fatigue, and safety conundrum in EMS. Prehosp Emerg Care 2012;16(4):572–6.

31. Chinoy ED, Cuellar JA, Huwa KE, et al. Performance of seven consumer sleep-tracking devices compared with polysomnography. Sleep 2021; 44(5).

32. Roberts DM, Schade MM, Mathew GM, et al. Detecting sleep using heart rate and motion data from multisensor consumer-grade wearables,

relative to wrist actigraphy and polysomnography. Sleep 2020;43(7).

33. Lee XK, Chee N, Ong JL, et al. Validation of a Consumer Sleep Wearable Device With Actigraphy and Polysomnography in Adolescents Across Sleep Opportunity Manipulations. J Clin Sleep Med 2019;15(9):1337–46.

34. Chinoy ED, Cuellar JA, Jameson JT, et al. Performance of Four Commercial Wearable Sleep-Tracking Devices Tested Under Unrestricted Conditions at Home in Healthy Young Adults. Nat Sci Sleep 2022;14:493–516.

35. Adler AB, Gunia BC, Bliese PD, et al. Using actigraphy feedback to improve sleep in soldiers: an exploratory trial. Sleep Health 2017;3(2):126–31.

36. Berryhill S, Morton CJ, Dean A, et al. Effect of wearables on sleep in healthy individuals: a randomized crossover trial and validation study. J Clin Sleep Med 2020;16(5):775–83.

37. Brunye TT, Yau K, Okano K, et al. Toward Predicting Human Performance Outcomes From Wearable Technologies: A Computational Modeling Approach. Front Physiol 2021;12:738973.

38. Perez-Pozuelo I, Zhai B, Palotti J, et al. The future of sleep health: a data-driven revolution in sleep science and medicine. NPJ Digit Med 2020;3:42.

39. Riedy SM, Fekedulegn D, Andrew M, et al. Generalizability of a biomathematical model of fatigue's sleep predictions. Chronobiol Int 2020;37(4): 564–72.

40. McCauley ME, McCauley P, Riedy SM, et al. Fatigue risk management based on self-reported fatigue: Expanding a biomathematical model of fatigue-related performance deficits to also predict subjective sleepiness. Transp Res Part F Traffic Psychol Behav 2021;79:94–106.

41. Hursh SR, Redmond DP, Johnson ML, et al. Fatigue models for applied research in warfighting. Aviat Space Environ Med 2004;75(3 Suppl):A44–53 [discussion: A54–60].

42. Reifman J, Kumar K, Hartman L, et al. 2B-Alert Web 2.0, an Open-Access Tool for Predicting Alertness and Optimizing the Benefits of Caffeine: Utility Study. J Med Internet Res 2022;24(1):e29595.

43. Rangan S, Riedy SM, Bassett R, et al. Predictive and proactive fatigue risk management approaches in commercial aviation. Chronobiol Int 2020;37(9–10):1479–82.

44. Dawson D, Ian Noy Y, Härmä M, et al. Modelling fatigue and the use of fatigue models in work settings. Accid Anal Prev 2011;43(2):549–64.

45. Caia J, Scott TJ, Halson SL, et al. The influence of sleep hygiene education on sleep in professional rugby league athletes. Sleep Health 2018;4(4): 364–8.

46. Fowler PM, Duffield R, Morrow I, et al. Effects of sleep hygiene and artificial bright light interventions on recovery from simulated international air travel. Eur J Appl Physiol 2015;115(3): 541–53.

47. Fowler PM, Knez W, Thornton HR, et al. Sleep Hygiene and Light Exposure Can Improve Performance Following Long-Haul Air Travel. Int J Sports Physiol Perform 2021;16(4):517–26.

48. Fullagar H, Skorski S, Duffield R, et al. The effect of an acute sleep hygiene strategy following a late-night soccer match on recovery of players. Chronobiol Int 2016;33(5):490–505.

49. Lever JR, Murphy AP, Duffield R, et al. A Combined Sleep Hygiene and Mindfulness Intervention to Improve Sleep and Well-Being During High-Performance Youth Tennis Tournaments. Int J Sports Physiol Perform 2021;16(2):250–8.

50. Harrison EM, Schmied EA, Hurtado SL, et al. The Development, Implementation, and Feasibility of a Circadian, Light, and Sleep Skills Program for Shipboard Military Personnel (CLASS-SM). Int J Environ Res Public Health 2022;19(5).

51. Bonnar D, Bartel K, Kakoschke N, et al. Sleep Interventions Designed to Improve Athletic Performance and Recovery: A Systematic Review of Current Approaches. Sports Med 2018;48(3): 683–703.

52. Albakri U, Drotos E, Meertens R. Sleep Health Promotion Interventions and Their Effectiveness: An Umbrella Review. Int J Environ Res Public Health 2021;18(11).

53. Rosekind n, Smith n, Miller n, et al. Alertness management: strategic naps in operational settings. J Sleep Res 1995;4(S2):62–6.

54. Lumley M, Roehrs T, Zorick F, et al. The alerting effects of naps in sleep-deprived subjects. Psychophysiology 1986;23(4):403–8.

55. Bonnet MH. The effect of varying prophylactic naps on performance, alertness and mood throughout a 52-hour continuous operation. Sleep 1991;14(4):307–15.

56. Rupp TL, Wesensten NJ, Bliese PD, et al. Banking sleep: realization of benefits during subsequent sleep restriction and recovery. Sleep 2009;32(3): 311–21.

57. Silva AC, Silva A, Edwards BJ, et al. Sleep extension in athletes: what we know so far - A systematic review. Sleep Med 2021;77:128–35.

58. Ritland BM, Simonelli G, Gentili RJ, et al. Effects of sleep extension on cognitive/motor performance and motivation in military tactical athletes. Sleep Med 2019;58:48–55.

59. Leduc C, Weaving D, Owen C, et al. The effect of acute sleep extension vs active recovery on post exercise recovery kinetics in rugby union players. PLoS One 2022;17(8):e0273026.

60. Mah CD, Mah KE, Kezirian EJ, et al. The effects of sleep extension on the athletic performance of

collegiate basketball players. Sleep 2011;34(7): 943–50.

61. Schwartz J, Simon RD Jr. Sleep extension improves serving accuracy: A study with college varsity tennis players. Physiol Behav 2015;151:541–4.

62. Arnal PJ, Lapole T, Erblang M, et al. Sleep Extension before Sleep Loss: Effects on Performance and Neuromuscular Function. Med Sci Sports Exerc 2016;48(8):1595–603.

63. Arnal PJ, Sauvet F, Leger D, et al. Benefits of Sleep Extension on Sustained Attention and Sleep Pressure Before and During Total Sleep Deprivation and Recovery. Sleep 2015;38(12):1935–43.

64. Lo JC, Koa TB, Ong JL, et al. Staying vigilant during recurrent sleep restriction: dose-response effects of time-in-bed and benefits of daytime napping. Sleep 2022;45(4).

65. Lastella M, Halson SL, Vitale JA, et al. To Nap or Not to Nap? A Systematic Review Evaluating Napping Behavior in Athletes and the Impact on Various Measures of Athletic Performance. Nat Sci Sleep 2021;13:841–62.

66. Boukhris O, Abdessalem R, Ammar A, et al. Nap Opportunity During the Daytime Affects Performance and Perceived Exertion in 5-m Shuttle Run Test. Front Physiol 2019;10:779.

67. Boukhris O, Trabelsi K, Ammar A, et al. A 90 min Daytime Nap Opportunity Is Better Than 40 min for Cognitive and Physical Performance. Int J Environ Res Public Health 2020;17(13).

68. Boukhris O, Trabelsi K, Ammar A, et al. Performance, muscle damage, and inflammatory responses to repeated high-intensity exercise following a 40-min nap. Res Sports Med 2021; 1–18.

69. Boukhris O, Trabelsi K, Hill DW, et al. Physiological response and physical performance after 40 min and 90 min daytime nap opportunities. Res Sports Med 2022;1–14.

70. Patterson PD, Weaver MD, Guyette FX, et al. Should public safety shift workers be allowed to nap while on duty? Am J Ind Med 2020;63(10): 843–50.

71. Hilditch CJ, McHill AW. Sleep inertia: current insights. Nat Sci Sleep 2019;11:155–65.

72. Centofanti S, Banks S, Coussens S, et al. A pilot study investigating the impact of a caffeine-nap on alertness during a simulated night shift. Chronobiol Int 2020;37(9–10):1469–73.

73. Hilditch CJ, Dorrian J, Banks S. Time to wake up: reactive countermeasures to sleep inertia. Ind Health 2016;54(6):528–41.

74. Hilditch CJ, Wong LR, Bathurst NG, et al. Rise and shine: The use of polychromatic short-wavelength-enriched light to mitigate sleep inertia at night following awakening from slow-wave sleep. J Sleep Res 2022;31(5):e13558.

75. Kamimori GH, McLellan TM, Tate CM, et al. Caffeine improves reaction time, vigilance and logical reasoning during extended periods with restricted opportunities for sleep. Psychopharmacology 2015;232(12):2031–42.

76. Killgore WD, Kamimori GH, Balkin TJ. Caffeine improves the efficiency of planning and sequencing abilities during sleep deprivation. J Clin Psychopharmacol 2014;34(5):660–2.

77. McLellan TM, Caldwell JA, Lieberman HR. A review of caffeine's effects on cognitive, physical and occupational performance. Neurosci Biobehav Rev 2016;71:294–312.

78. McLellan TM, Kamimori GH, Bell DG, et al. Caffeine maintains vigilance and marksmanship in simulated urban operations with sleep deprivation. Aviat Space Environ Med 2005;76(1):39–45.

79. McLellan TM, Kamimori GH, Voss DM, et al. Caffeine maintains vigilance and improves run times during night operations for Special Forces. Aviat Space Environ Med 2005;76(7):647–54.

80. Ramakrishnan S, Laxminarayan S, Wesensten NJ, et al. Dose-dependent model of caffeine effects on human vigilance during total sleep deprivation. J Theor Biol 2014;358:11–24.

81. Doty TJ, So CJ, Bergman EM, et al. Limited efficacy of caffeine and recovery costs during and following 5 days of chronic sleep restriction. Sleep 2017; 40(12). https://doi.org/10.1093/sleep/zsx171.

82. Guest NS, VanDusseldorp TA, Nelson MT, et al. International society of sports nutrition position stand: caffeine and exercise performance. J Int Soc Sports Nutr 2021;18(1):1.

83. Priezjev NV, Vital-Lopez FG, Reifman J. Assessment of the unified model of performance: accuracy of group-average and individualised alertness predictions. J Sleep Res 2022;e13626.

84. Dornbierer DA, Yerlikaya F, Wespi R, et al. A novel bedtime pulsatile-release caffeine formula ameliorates sleep inertia symptoms immediately upon awakening. Sci Rep 2021;11(1):19734.

85. Romdhani M, Souissi N, Moussa-Chamari I, et al. Caffeine Use or Napping to Enhance Repeated Sprint Performance After Partial Sleep Deprivation: Why Not Both? Int J Sports Physiol Perform 2021; 16(5):711–8.

86. Vandewalle G, Maquet P, Dijk DJ. Light as a modulator of cognitive brain function. Trends Cogn Sci 2009;13(10):429–38.

87. Fernandez FX. Current Insights into Optimal Lighting for Promoting Sleep and Circadian Health: Brighter Days and the Importance of Sunlight in the Built Environment. Nat Sci Sleep 2022;14: 25–39.

88. Figueiro MG, Pedler D. Red light: A novel, non-pharmacological intervention to promote alertness in shift workers. J Safety Res 2020;74:169–77.

89. Guarana CL, Barnes CM, Ong WJ. The effects of blue-light filtration on sleep and work outcomes. J Appl Psychol 2021;106(5):784–96.

90. Sletten TL, Raman B, Magee M, et al. A Blue-Enriched, Increased Intensity Light Intervention to Improve Alertness and Performance in Rotating Night Shift Workers in an Operational Setting. Nat Sci Sleep 2021;13:647–57.

91. Janse van Rensburg DCC, Jansen van Rensburg A, Fowler P, et al. How to manage travel fatigue and jet lag in athletes? A systematic review of interventions. Br J Sports Med 2020;54(16):960–8.

92. Roach GD, Sargent C. Interventions to Minimize Jet Lag After Westward and Eastward Flight. Front Physiol 2019;10:927.

93. Zhou Y, Chen Q, Luo X, et al. Does Bright Light Counteract the Post-lunch Dip in Subjective States and Cognitive Performance Among Undergraduate Students? Front Public Health 2021;9:652849.

94. Figueiro MG, Sahin L, Roohan C, et al. Effects of red light on sleep inertia. Nat Sci Sleep 2019;11:45–57.

95. Slama H, Deliens G, Schmitz R, et al. Afternoon nap and bright light exposure improve cognitive flexibility post lunch. PLoS One 2015;10(5):e0125359.

96. Wilckens KA, Ferrarelli F, Walker MP, et al. Slow-Wave Activity Enhancement to Improve Cognition. Trends Neurosci 2018;41(7):470–82.

97. Luber B, Lisanby SH. Enhancement of human cognitive performance using transcranial magnetic stimulation (TMS). Neuroimage 2014;85(Pt 3):961–70.

98. Luber B, Stanford AD, Bulow P, et al. Remediation of sleep-deprivation-induced working memory impairment with fMRI-guided transcranial magnetic stimulation. Cereb Cortex 2008;18(9):2077–85.

99. Luber B, Steffener J, Tucker A, et al. Extended remediation of sleep deprived-induced working memory deficits using fMRI-guided transcranial magnetic stimulation. Sleep 2013;36(6):857–71.

100. McIntire LK, McKinley RA, Goodyear C, et al. A comparison of the effects of transcranial direct current stimulation and caffeine on vigilance and cognitive performance during extended wakefulness. Brain Stimul 2014;7(4):499–507.

101. McIntire LK, McKinley RA, Nelson JM, et al. Transcranial direct current stimulation versus caffeine as a fatigue countermeasure. Brain Stimul 2017;10(6):1070–8.

102. Bellesi M, Riedner BA, Garcia-Molina GN, et al. Enhancement of sleep slow waves: underlying mechanisms and practical consequences. Front Syst Neurosci 2014;8:208.

103. Huber R, Esser SK, Ferrarelli F, et al. TMS-induced cortical potentiation during wakefulness locally increases slow wave activity during sleep. PLoS One 2007;2(3):e276.

104. Huber R, Maatta S, Esser SK, et al. Measures of cortical plasticity after transcranial paired associative stimulation predict changes in electroencephalogram slow-wave activity during subsequent sleep. J Neurosci 2008;28(31):7911–8.

105. Massimini M, Ferrarelli F, Esser SK, et al. Triggering sleep slow waves by transcranial magnetic stimulation. Proc Natl Acad Sci U S A 2007;104(20):8496–501.

106. Stefanou MI, Baur D, Belardinelli P, et al. Brain State-dependent Brain Stimulation with Real-time Electroencephalography-Triggered Transcranial Magnetic Stimulation. J Vis Exp 2019;(150). https://doi.org/10.3791/59711.

107. Marshall L, Kirov R, Brade J, et al. Transcranial electrical currents to probe EEG brain rhythms and memory consolidation during sleep in humans. PLoS One 2011;6(2):e16905.

108. Reato D, Gasca F, Datta A, et al. Transcranial electrical stimulation accelerates human sleep homeostasis. PLoS Comput Biol 2013;9(2):e1002898.

109. Marshall L, Helgadottir H, Molle M, et al. Boosting slow oscillations during sleep potentiates memory. Nature 2006;444(7119):610–3.

110. Marshall L, Molle M, Hallschmid M, et al. Transcranial direct current stimulation during sleep improves declarative memory. J Neurosci 2004;24(44):9985–92.

111. Malkani RG, Zee PC. Brain Stimulation for Improving Sleep and Memory. Sleep Med Clin 2020;15(1):101–15.

112. Huber R, Ghilardi MF, Massimini M, et al. Arm immobilization causes cortical plastic changes and locally decreases sleep slow wave activity. Nat Neurosci 2006;9(9):1169–76.

113. Huber R, Ghilardi MF, Massimini M, et al. Local sleep and learning. Nature 2004;430(6995):78–81.

114. Navarrete M, Schneider J, Ngo HV, et al. Examining the optimal timing for closed-loop auditory stimulation of slow-wave sleep in young and older adults. Sleep 2020;43(6).

115. Ngo HV, Martinetz T, Born J, et al. Auditory closed-loop stimulation of the sleep slow oscillation enhances memory. Neuron 2013;78(3):545–53.

116. Ngo HV, Miedema A, Faude I, et al. Driving sleep slow oscillations by auditory closed-loop stimulation-a self-limiting process. J Neurosci 2015;35(17):6630–8.

117. Diep C, Ftouni S, Manousakis JE, et al. Acoustic slow wave sleep enhancement via a novel,

automated device improves executive function in middle-aged men. Sleep 2020;43(1).

118. Sousouri G, Krugliakova E, Skorucak J, et al. Neuromodulation by means of phase-locked auditory stimulation affects key marker of excitability and connectivity during sleep. Sleep 2022;45(1).

119. Papalambros NA, Santostasi G, Malkani RG, et al. Acoustic Enhancement of Sleep Slow Oscillations and Concomitant Memory Improvement in Older Adults. Front Hum Neurosci 2017;11:109.

120. Cordi MJ, Rasch B. How robust are sleep-mediated memory benefits? Curr Opin Neurobiol 2021; 67:1–7.

A 2022 Survey of Commercially Available Smartphone Apps for Sleep
Most Enhance Sleep

Tracy Jill Doty, PhD[a],*, Emily K. Stekl, BA[a], Matthew Bohn, BS[a],
Grace Klosterman, BS[a], Guido Simonelli, MD[a,b,c], Jacob Collen, MD[d,e]

KEYWORDS

- mHealth - Reduced sleep latency - Consumer sleep technology - Mobile technology
- Sleep tracker

KEY POINTS

- Most sleep apps available to consumers are designed to enhance sleep by reducing sleep latency with auditory stimuli.
- While most sleep apps do not have peer-reviewed evidence supporting the specific app, most do use types of enhancement that are backed by scientific evidence.
- Sleep apps are widely available, low to no cost, and mostly focus on helping the consumer fall sleep faster using sounds.
- Sleep apps could be considered a possible strategy for patients and consumers to improve their sleep, although more validation of these apps is recommended.

INTRODUCTION

While sufficient and quality sleep is critical for health,[1] chronic sleep loss is strikingly pervasive within the global population.[2,3] In addition to the negative health impact on an individual, chronic sleep loss is also a costly problem for society. In the U.S. alone it is estimated that $411 billion is lost every year due to insufficient sleep.[4] Also within the U.S., more individuals are seeking treatment for sleep disorders.[5] Moreover, globally the problem of chronic sleep loss and insomnia appears to have grown during the COVID-19 pandemic.[6,7]

As the global epidemic of sleep loss continues to increase, and concerns about the dangers of sleep loss grow, the demand for Sleep Medicine specialty care has risen. The COVID-19 pandemic only worsened these concerns, as health-related fears and even greater limitations in access to outpatient care were amplified. The COVID-19 virus itself has been linked to a rise in insomnia.[8,9] Unfortunately, there is a widespread shortage of Sleep providers. Some estimates hold that across the U.S., one Sleep physician could be empaneled with over 40,000 patients per provider.[10] The limitless potential of the online environment has given rise to a boom in telehealth.[11] Previously the domain of behavioral health and numerous other specialties have come to realize that telemedicine has the benefits of safety and social distancing,

[a] Behavioral Biology Branch, Walter Reed Army Institute of Research, 503 Robert Grant Avenue, Silver Spring, MD 20910, USA; [b] Departments of Medicine and Neuroscience, Faculty of Medicine, Université de Montréal, 5400 Boulevard Gouin Ouest (Office J-5000), Montréal, QC H4J 1C5, Canada; [c] Centre d'études vancées en médecine du sommeil, Hôpital du Sacré-Coeur de Montréal, Montréal, CIUSSS du Nord de l'Île-de-Montréal, 5400 Boulevard Gouin Ouest (Office J-5000), Montréal, QC H4J 1C5, Canada; [d] Department of Medicine, Uniformed Services University of the Health Sciences, 4301 Jones Bridge Road, Bethesda, MD 20814, USA; [e] Pulmonary, Critical Care and Sleep Medicine, Walter Reed National Military Medical Center, 8901 Rockville Pike, Bethesda, MD 20889, USA
* Corresponding author.
E-mail address: tracy.j.doty2.civ@health.mil

Sleep Med Clin 18 (2023) 373–384
https://doi.org/10.1016/j.jsmc.2023.05.008
1556-407X/23/Published by Elsevier Inc. This is an open access article under the CC BY-NC-ND license (http://creativecommons.org/licenses/by-nc-nd/4.0/).

reducing the need for brick-and-mortar facilities, reducing foot traffic and parking demands, and increasing efficiency. Unfortunately, although more convenient for patients, telemedicine still requires the same amount of a provider's time, and the ability to bill for services is limited. Digital prescription therapy for addiction and insomnia has emerged, yet these are also costly services that may be difficult to access.

The virtual environment continues to demonstrate its agility with respect to consumer health demands with an unheralded rise in health-related smartphone apps also known as mobile health (mHealth) apps. A 2021 report from the IQVIA Institute for Human Data Science noted that 90,000 new consumer health apps were introduced in 2020 leading to over 350,000 health apps available to consumers by the end of 2020.[12] As more mHealth apps are available to the consumer, more consumers are also using smartphones. The Pew Research Center estimated that as of February 2021, 85% of American adults owned a smartphone, up from 35% in May of 2011.[13]

A growing sector of health-related smartphone apps are apps focused on sleep - an example of a Consumer Sleep Technology (CST) as defined by the American Academy of Sleep Medicine (AASM).[14] In the AASM's 2018 statement on CSTs, it is recognized that "Most CSTs are not FDA cleared or validated clinical devices/applications, but widespread accessibility and use by patients (and potential patients) may augment patient engagement." The statement also notes other potential advantages of CSTs such as popularity and low cost.

While the number of health-related smartphone apps and smartphone users continues to increase, there does not appear to be a recent complete review of sleep-related smartphone apps available to consumers. Largely, previous reviews of sleep smartphone apps have focused on apps that measure sleep.[15–20] A focus on the measurement of sleep also appears within the broader context of consumer sleep-related technology to include wearable and mobile technology as noted within a scoping review.[21] Additional reviews have included only consumer apps related to sleep problems broadly[22] or specifically, such as for obstructive sleep apnea.[23]

Additionally, there is little to no literature centered on the number of sleep-related smartphone apps that aim to enhance or improve sleep. In fact, these types of apps have been specifically removed from other global reviews of sleep apps available on the consumer market. For example, a 2018 review excluded 642 "environmental sound/meditation/relaxation" apps from a review

of apps that support sleep self-management, although this category of apps accounted for over a fourth of all sleep apps found in the initial review.[20]

With the recent increase of sleep technology on the market, it can be difficult for consumers and healthcare providers to understand the scope and utility of what is available. Previous sleep-related health app surveys have focused almost exclusively on sleep measurement. However, to our knowledge, no efforts have been made to systematically identify all existing apps in the consumer market, and the main characteristics of these devices (ie, when and how they are used). We sought to identify existing consumer sleep apps and provide a comprehensive review of the main characteristics of these apps, and look into the types of evidence (if any) the developers offered to supports their claims.

METHODS/APPROACH
Search Strategy

Both the Android Google Play Store and the Apple iOS App Store were searched on 26SEP2022 in Maryland, U.S. Google and Apple restrict store browsing on devices that are not compatible with the download and use of their proprietary applications, so instead of searching their store websites on a search engine such as Google Chrome, alternative platforms were used to conduct the search. A Google Chromebook was used to search the Google Play Store and the iOS App Store was searched using two third-party websites linked to the store (https://theappstore.org/and https://fnd.io/), in addition to searching the store on an iPhone 12. Store searches were conducted by entering the keyword "sleep" into the search bars of each platform. Results from the Google Play Store and the two websites linked to the iOS App Store were exported to PDFs. The iPhone 12 search was used as a quality check to confirm that the apps found in the website searches were inclusive of all Apple apps offered on the iOS App Store. As Google Play Store apps function on the Android mobile operating system platform, apps found within the Google Play Store are referred to as Android apps throughout the rest of this article.

Inclusion and Exclusion Criteria

Two reviewers independently assessed the smartphone applications identified from the search. We included any application related to sleep or sleep processes, such as sleep initiation and maintenance, sleep hygiene, sleep behavior, and wake after sleep. We excluded non-sleep-related apps, which included apps that used "sleep" as a hashtag or as a word in their description to gain more search hits but that did not have features related to sleep. Examples included games, voice changers, and Christmas countdown timer apps.

Data Extraction

One reviewer extracted data from the iOS App Store results and one reviewer extracted data from the Google Play Store results. Both reviewers quality checked the data from both stores for accuracy following extraction. Data extraction fields were determined through an iterative process. Following the inclusion and exclusion determination, specific app data was extracted from the description and screenshots provided by the seller. Basic app information was collected first and included: the name of the application; the seller of the app; the store (Apple or Android) where the app was identified; and whether the application could be found on both Apple and Android platforms. In addition, another extraction column was added to note if the app had been identified in our previous 2021 survey,[24] that was conducted in June and July 2021 using a similar search strategy as the one described above.

Next, reviewers extracted relevant sleep-related data. Starting with sleep app type, apps were sorted into one of the 6 sleep app types: sleep enhancement, sleep measurement, both enhancement and measurement, snore detection, manual trackers, and basic alarms. Basic alarms included standard alarm clocks; manual trackers included those that required manual logging of bed and wake times; and snore detection was those using the phone microphone to record snoring and talking during sleep. Sleep measurement apps included the use of accelerometry, microphones, or paired devices to directly measure sleep stages, heart rate, or other physiological measures during sleep. Sleep enhancement apps included an attempt to reduce sleep latency, the use of a smart alarm to reduce sleep inertia upon awakening, or apps that provided sleep hygiene programs or access to sleep coaches for personalized sleep improvement insights.

The sleep enhancement app types had further data extracted regarding the methods used to reduce sleep latency. These apps were categorized as using either visual or auditory stimuli to target sleep latency; and auditory stimuli were further broken down to: Verbal stimuli (bedtime stories; guided meditations; or lyrical music) and Nonverbal stimuli (nature sounds; artificial sounds including white noise and binaural beats; and instrumental music).

Additional extraction fields included cost information: free version available; subscription or one-time payment option available; and subscription or one-time payment amount. Lastly, whether the apps were designed to be used during wake or sleep was determined; and whether there was peer-reviewed evidence to support the sleep claims the apps were making.

Data Analysis

Descriptive statistics on the collected app data were performed using SPSS Version 25. Frequencies of categories were assessed for all sleep-related apps and then the data were further broken down to include only apps utilizing Enhancement (eg, those apps labeled as "Enhancement Only" or "Both" for the Sleep App Type category) and only apps utilizing Measurement (eg, those apps labeled as "Measurement Only" or "Both" for the Sleep App Type category). Enhancement apps were further broken down to only assess frequencies with the Reduced Sleep Latency apps (eg, those apps labeled as "Reduced Sleep Latency, Reduced Sleep Latency and Sleep Hygiene Tips", "Reduced Sleep Latency and Smart Alarm", or "Reduced Sleep Latency and Sleep Hygiene Tips and Smart Alarm" for the Enhancement App Type category). Furthermore, while descriptive statistics were assessed for sleep-related apps as a whole, all data were also split and compared by App Store.

RESULTS
Overall App Information

Of the 512 apps that appeared in both the Google Play and Apple App Stores searching with the keyword "sleep," 461 were deemed to be truly sleep-related. **Table 1** and **Fig. 1** outline descriptive statistics for all apps. Of the 461 apps, 270 (58.6%) were also found in a 2021 survey conducted using the same method and 192 (41.6%) were apps of the same name found in both app stores. A large majority of all apps had a free version available (N = 422, 95.9%) and the cost per app ranged from $0.00 to $119.99, with the average cost per app being $9.77± $17.31 (standard deviation). While most apps offer at least a free trial version, only 120 (26%) remained free and had no payment options. Over half of the apps had a subscription option (N = 242, 52.5%) and 21.5% had a one-time purchase option (N = 99).

The large majority of apps were designed to be used during wake (N = 354, 76.8%), 13.0% (N = 60) were designed to be used both during sleep and wake, and only 10.2% (N = 47) during sleep alone. Only 18 apps (3.9%) had peer-reviewed evidence using the specific app. These apps are discussed in more detail later in

Table 1
All commercially available sleep apps found in both the android and apple app stores

		All Sleep Apps		
		Both Stores N = 461	Android N = 233 (50.5% of total)	Apple N = 228 (49.5.% of total)
In 2021 Survey		270 (58.6%)	101 (43.3%)	169 (74.1%)
In Both App Stores		192 (41.6%)	73 (31.3%)	119 (52.2%)
Free Version Available		442 (95.9%)	229 (98.3%)	213 (93.4%)
Cost Range		$0.00–119.99	$0.00–119.99	$0.00–119.99
Average Cost (±sd)		$9.77 ± $17.31	$6.18 ± $14.27	$13.48 ± $19.30
Payment Option	Free – No Payment Options	120 (26.0%)	91 (39.1%)	29 (12.7%)
	Onetime	99 (21.5%)	47 (20.2%)	52 (22.8%)
	Subscription	242 (52.5%)	95 (40.8%)	147 (64.5%)
When is App Used?	Sleep	47 (10.2%)	18 (7.7%)	29 (12.7%)
	Wake	354 (76.8%)	188 (80.7%)	166 (72.8%)
	Both	60 (13.0%)	27 (11.6%)	33 (14.5%)
Peer-Reviewed Evidence for Specific App Exists		18 (3.9%)	7 (3.0%)	11 (4.8%)
Type of App	Enhancement Only	338 (73.3%)	183 (78.5%)	155 (68.0%)
	Measurement Only	22 (4.8%)	3 (1.3%)	19 (8.3%)
	Both Measurement and Enhancement	57 (12.4%)	24 (10.3%)	33 (14.5%)
	Manual Tracker	29 (6.3%)	16 (6.9%)	13 (5.7%)
	Snore Detection	8 (1.7%)	5 (2.1%)	3 (1.3%)
	Basic Alarm	7 (1.5%)	2 (0.9%)	5 (2.2%)

discussion. Most apps were labeled "Enhancement Only" in this survey (N = 338, 73.3%), 22 were labeled "Measurement Only" (4.8%), and 57 used both Measurement and Enhancement (12.4%). Less than 10% of apps fell into the final three categories: Manual Tracker (N = 29, 6.3%), Snore Detection (N = 8, 1.7%), and Basic Alarm (N = 7, 1.5%).

Enhancement Apps

Descriptive statistics for Enhancement Apps can be found in **Table 2** and **Fig. 1** and account for all apps categorized as utilizing enhancement (N = 395, 85.7% of all sleep-related apps) – including those apps categorized as both enhancement and measurement. For these apps, descriptive statistics were like the overall statistics found in **Table 1**. As for the method of enhancement, most apps utilized reduced sleep latency (N = 370, 93.7%). Only 25 apps did not utilize some form of reduced sleep latency; these included Sleep Hygiene Tips or Program (N = 20, 5.1%) and Smart Alarms (N = 5, 1.3%). These Enhancement Apps were further examined

for the type of reduced sleep latency they utilized (**Fig. 2**). We found that the large majority of Enhancement Apps used auditory stimuli alone (N = 311, 78.7%). When these apps were further parsed out, it was found that most apps used non-verbal stimuli either exclusively (N = 176, 48.4%) or in concert with verbal stimuli (N = 151, 41.5%). Apps tended to use a variety of verbal and non-verbal stimuli, often even within a single app; therefore, all types of auditory stimuli are reported here as overlapping categories. Apps using verbal stimuli relied most heavily on Guided Meditation (N = 142, 75.5%), but also used Stories (N = 101, 53.7%) and Lyrical Music (N = 44, 23.4%). Apps using non-verbal stimuli used Nature Sounds (N = 286, 87.5%) and Instrumental Music (N = 239, 73.1%) most frequently and Artificial Sounds, such as binaural beats, were used less often (N = 70, 21.4%).

It is worth noting that all but four of the apps with peer-reviewed evidence were Enhancement Apps (N = 14, 3.5% of all Enhancement Apps). Two Enhancement Apps found in both App Stores that have several peer-reviewed studies evaluating the app are Calm (eg,[25–27]) and Headspace

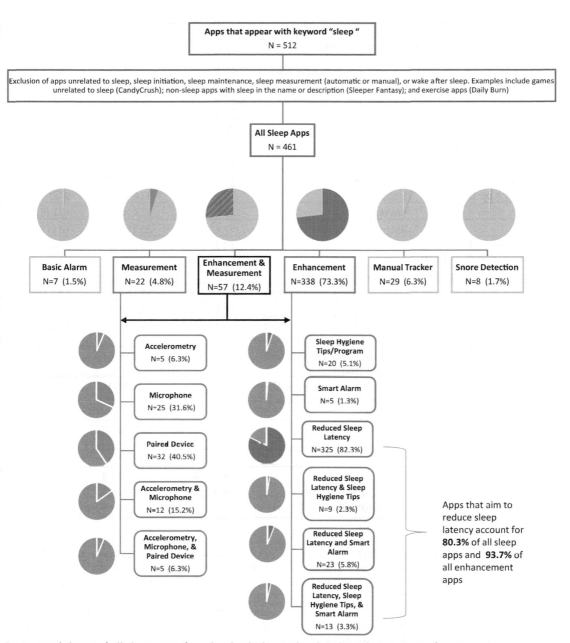

Fig. 1. Breakdown of all sleep apps found in both the Android and Apple App Stores by use.

(eg,[28–30]). A recent systematic review of studies investigating both apps concluded that Headspace had more randomized trials associated with it and the results were promising.[31] Both these apps aimed to reduce sleep latency with both verbal and non-verbal auditory stimulation applied before sleep.

Measurement Apps

Measurement Apps accounted for less than 20% of all commercially available sleep apps (N = 79, 17.1% of all apps; **Table 3**). In contrast to

Enhancement Apps, Measurement Apps were primarily designed to use during Sleep only (N = 29, 36.7%) or during both Sleep and Wake (N = 50, 63.3% - many apps used for both enhancement and measurement fell into this category). Forty percent of Measurement Apps were paired to a device only (N = 32), 31.6% used a microphone only (N = 25), and 6.3% used accelerometry only (6.3%). Some combined accelerometry with a microphone (N = 12, 15.2%), while a few others used all three methods (N = 5, 6.3%).

Eight Measurement Apps had peer-reviewed research associated with the app. Seven of those

Table 2
All commercially available sleep apps that focus on enhancement

Enhancement Apps		Both Stores	Android	Apple
Total		395	207 (52.4%)	188 (47.6%)
In 2021 Survey		232 (58.7%)	91 (44.0%)	141 (75%)
In Both App Stores		165 (41.8%)	68 (32.9%)	97 (51.6%)
Free Version Available		381 (96.5%)	203 (98.1%)	178 (94.7%)
Cost Range		$0.00–119.99	$0.00–119.99	$0.00–99.99
When is App Used?	Sleep	13 (3.3%)	9 (4.3%)	4 (2.1%)
	Wake	325 (82.3%)	173 (83.6%)	152 (80.9%)
	Both	57 (14.4%)	25 (12.1%)	32 (17.0%)
Peer-Reviewed Evidence for Specific App Exists		14 (3.5%)	5 (2.4%)	9 (4.8%)
Enhancement Method	Reduced Sleep Latency	325 (82.3%)	168 (81.2%)	157 (83.5%)
	Sleep Hygiene Tips/Program	20 (5.1%)	16 (7.7%)	4 (2.1%)
	Smart Alarm	5 (1.3%)	2 (1.0%)	3 (1.6%)
	Reduced Sleep Latency and Sleep Hygiene Tips/Program	9 (2.3%)	5 (2.4%)	4 (2.1%)
	Reduced Sleep Latency and Smart Alarm	23 (5.8%)	10 (4.8%)	13 (6.9%)
	Reduced Sleep Latency, Sleep Hygiene Tips, and Smart Alarm	13 (3.3%)	6 (2.9%)	7 (3.7%)
Type of Reduced Sleep Latency Enhancement	Auditory	311 (78.7%)	166 (80.2%)	145 (77.1%)
	Visual	6 (1.5%)	5 (2.4%)	1 (0.5%)
	Both	53 (13.4%)	18 (8.7%)	35 (18.6%)
	None (does not utilize Reduced Sleep Latency)	25 (6.3%)	18 (8.7%)	7 (3.7%)

apps utilized a paired device: Fitbit,[32,33] Sleep-tracker – AI,[34] Oura,[35,36] SleepSpace – Tracker & Coach,[37] Withings Health Mate,[38] Sleep as Android: Smart alarm,[20] and Nanit.[39] Sleep Cycle AB utilized the microphone and accelerometry on the phone instead of a paired device and also had peer-reviewed data published on its use.[40]

Android Versus Apple

The types of sleep apps available to the consumer are similar between the Android and Apple App Stores with a few exceptions. First, Android had a greater turnover of apps from 2021 to 2022. While 74.1% of Apple apps were found in the 2021 survey, only 43.3% of Android apps were. Second, Android provided more apps with free versions (Android = 229, 98.4% vs Apple = 213, 93.4%) and the average cost of an app was less (Android = $6.18 ± $14.27, Apple = $13.48 ± $19.30). Third, Apple offers more Subscription

options but less apps that are completely free without payment necessary (Subscription: Android = 95, Apple = 147; Totally Free: Android = 91, Apple = 29). Lastly, Apple did have more Measurement Apps available (Android = 27, Apple = 52) and seven of the eight Measurement Apps with peer-reviewed evidence were available from Apple.

DISCUSSION

The high number of consumer health-related smartphone apps and consumers using smartphone apps means that individuals have access to a potentially wide variety of mobile technology. In this global review of commercially available sleep apps, we found over 400 apps across both the Android and Apple platforms. Notably, the large majority were enhancement apps that aimed to reduce sleep latency before bed using sounds. It is interesting that while the majority of sleep apps

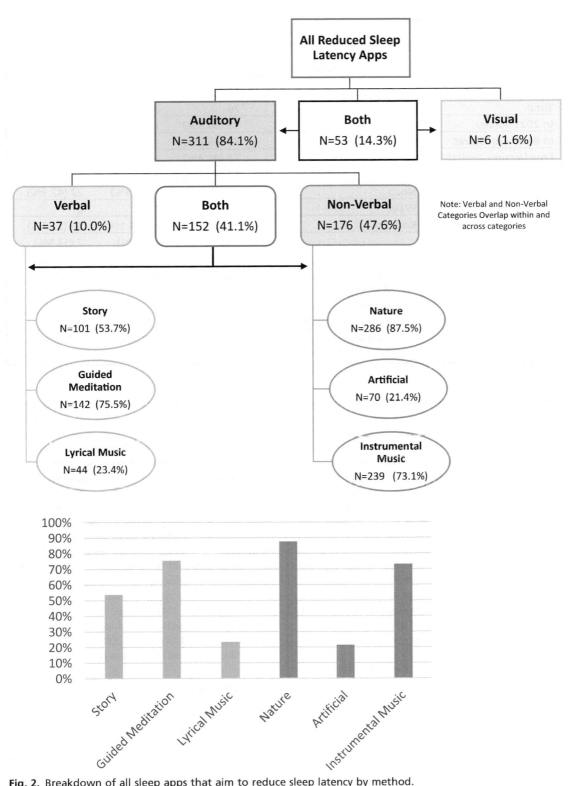

Fig. 2. Breakdown of all sleep apps that aim to reduce sleep latency by method.

Table 3
All commercially available apps that focus on measurement

Measurement Apps		Both Stores	Android	Apple
Total		79	27 (34.2%)	52 (65.8%)
In 2021 Survey		48 (60.8%)	11 (40.7%)	37 (71.2%)
In Both App Stores		39 (49.4%)	11 (40.7%)	28 (53.8%)
Free Version Available		73 (92.4%)	27 (100%)	46 (88.5%)
Cost Range		$0.00–119.99	$0.00–119.99	$0.00–119.99
When is App Used?	Sleep	29 (36.7%)	7 (25.9%)	22 (42.3%)
	Wake	0	0	0
	Both	50 (63.3%)	20 (74.1%)	30 (57.7%)
Peer-Reviewed Evidence for Specific App Exists		8 (10.1%)	1 (3.7%)	7 (13.5%)
Measurement Method	Microphone	25 (31.6%)	11 (40.7%)	14 (26.9%)
	Paired Device	32 (40.5%)	6 (22.2%)	26 (50.0%)
	Accelerometry	5 (6.3%)	3 (11.1%)	2 (3.8%)
	Accelerometry and Microphone	12 (15.2%)	5 (18.5%)	7 (13.5%)
	Accelerometry, Microphone, and Paired Device	5 (6.3%)	2 (7.4%)	3 (5.8%)

available to the consumer focus on the enhancement of sleep, the majority of the reviews and peer-reviewed evidence for sleep apps focus on sleep measurement. This sheds light on an important area of future research and review.

Most apps were designed to be used during wake rather than during sleep. On the surface, this may seem paradoxical but as most apps were utilized to shorten time to fall asleep, they were only designed to be used in the waking period before sleep. Those apps designed to be used during sleep were primarily measurement apps. Also, most apps had a free version available so that a consumer could test an app out without having to purchase a subscription or the app itself. Sleep apps were evenly split across the two apps stores with roughly 40% apps being the same app found in both stores.

Compared to our 2021 survey of sleep apps, over 58% of apps were new for 2022. This may represent a rapid turnover in apps available. For the consumer or patient this may mean access to newer content more frequently but also the consumer or patient may lose access to apps that they have found particularly valuable to use. It is worth noting that this turnover was higher for Android compared to Apple apps (43.3% vs 74.1%).

Only a handful of apps had been evaluated within peer-reviewed publications, however, the broad use of auditory stimulation to reduce sleep latency has been proven to be effective in a multitude of studies. There is evidence to support the use of verbal stimuli such as Guided Meditation[41] and Lyrical Music.[42] There is also evidence to support the use of Non-Verbal Stimuli such as Nature sounds,[43] Artificial sounds,[44] and Instrumental Music[42] in helping people fall sleep faster.

While the majority of sleep apps focus on enhancement, there are some measurement apps on the market. More of these apps have peer-reviewed evidence support and many are used with a paired device. Recent validation work suggests that at least some of these sleep measurement devices with associated smartphone apps do a reasonably good job of measuring total sleep time.[32] Therefore, it is important to consider that at least some of these apps with paired devices could provide relevant information for sleep medicine providers.[45]

LIMITATIONS

A limitation of this work is that it is only a survey of commercially available sleep apps on a given day. It does not capture how many users downloaded these apps, how often they are used, or how highly they are rated by users. Additionally, we did not assess or appraise the apps in this survey. There are rating tools available such as the Mobile Application Rating System (MARS) quality score.[46] These tools allow researchers to directly compare apps and provide recommendations, but they are also time-consuming to utilize for a large cohort such as this global review. Given that over 40% of commercially available sleep apps available in 2021 were not available in 2020 in our survey, it may not make sense to invest in the assessment and appraisal of all sleep apps. Finally, we only surveyed commercially available apps found in the Android and Apple App Stores using "sleep" as a search word. There are other sleep apps available in other App Stores as well as apps that only a select group of users have access to such as prescription only apps, beta testing apps, and apps only available directly from a company and not through the app store. Prescription sleep apps represent a growing market that includes digital Cognitive Behavior Therapy for Insomnia (CBT-i) as well as apps associated with prescribed devices such as CPAPs.

It is unavoidable that medical providers will be called upon to answer patients' questions about these apps. Although sleep apps have the potential to raise awareness about sleep, improve sleep quality, and access to care, they could paradoxically increase patient preoccupation with sleep, or even generate new, and unexpected, anxieties surrounding sleep.

Physicians will need to be prepared for patients to request guidance regarding sleep apps. This can place physicians in a difficult situation clinically and ethically. Physicians are credentialed to provide evidence-based, subject matter expertise on diagnosing and treating clinical disorders. The use of sleep apps to treat a sleep disorder, such as insomnia, as opposed to simply improve wellness, is quite different. Patients are unlikely to appreciate that there are differences between clinical care for medical disorders and augmenting wellness and performance. Diagnosis and treatment of a disorder is very different than guidance aimed at improving lifestyle, quality of life, and athletic performance.

Physicians are entrusted by the public to provide medical care, but not to endorse a commercial product. Ethical quandaries could arise with physicians that create their own sleep apps which they market to patients. Ethical conflicts of interest could diminish physician credibility, and even damage patient confidence in conservative treatments for sleep disorders (ie, the potential for patients to be influenced by a bad experience with a sleep app when considering digital CBT-i).

However, physicians should start to build some literacy about sleep apps. These interventions are here to stay and building a basic understanding of available products and having some rehearsed guidance for patients can reduce confusion and the potential for distracting and frustrating discussions with patients during office visits.

Future research that quantifies the efficacy of sleep apps is needed to fill the gap in the literature that we have identified. However, the multidisciplinary nature of sleep medical care and the wide-ranging impact of commercially available sleep apps would be best served with mixed methods research, particularly qualitative evaluations using feedback from key stakeholders (patients, bed partners, and physicians), to catch up to an industry that has a huge head start over clinicians.

CLINICS CARE POINTS

Products: What do They do?

- Sleep apps are versatile, can be used anywhere, do not require physician engagement or a prescription.
- There are many apps available across both Android and Apple platforms and most have a free version available
- Most sleep apps target the enhancement of sleep by playing auditory stimuli before sleep
- Commercially available sleep apps represent a potentially valuable opportunity for patients to try out free apps that may help reduce sleep latency with sounds

The patient (and their bed partner): How can these devices impact the bedroom, intimacy, and family?

- There is significant potential for patients to benefit from sleep apps, given ease of use, low cost, volume, and variety. Benefits might be expected to include:
  - Greater sense of control over their sleep
  - Greater insight regarding their own sleep
  - Avoidance of medication side effects, or even side effects of cognitive behavioral interventions such as sleep restriction or sleep compression
  - Cost savings
- Harms are limited and unlikely but may include unwarranted anxiety surrounding sleep, or the potential for auditory stimuli in apps to paradoxically disrupt sleep.
- There is no evidence regarding how sleep apps are perceived by, or affect the sleep of, a patient's bedpartner. Any intervention that unintentionally improves the sleep of the patient at the expense of the bedpartner can have unseen consequences for other individuals and the patient's relationship with their partner.

- Unfortunately, most of these apps have not been validated with peer-reviewed evidence, but most do utilize techniques that have been validated.

Physician: Awareness, Knowledge, and Preparation

- Physicians may be asked to interpret data from apps, or patient questions regarding apps, that falls outside the standards of evidence-based medicine.
- Physicians must begin to understand and be able to articulate, the differences between:
  - Telemedicine
  - Commercial sleep technologies, including digital wearables
  - Sleep apps, including smartphone apps designed to enhance sleep
  - Home sleep testing
  - FDA approved Digital prescription therapeutics (such as *Somryst* for insomnia, or *Nightware* , for nightmare disorder)
- Physicians should start to consider crafting their own disclaimers or internal policies for handling patient queries. Setting boundaries on these conversations (in both time and content) may improve the doctor-patient relationship and reduce time and distractions during clinical visits.
- Physicians should consider ethical and professional standards with regards to boundaries between diagnosing and treating medical disorders and endorsing commercial products aimed at improving health and wellness.

DISCLAIMER

Material has been reviewed by the Walter Reed Army Institute of Research. There is no objection to its presentation and/or publication. The opinions or assertions contained herein are the private views of the author, and are not to be construed as official, or as reflecting true views of the Department of the Army or the Department of Defense.

DISCLOSURE

The authors have no commercial or financial conflicts of interest to report.

SUPPORT

Support for this study came from the Department of Defense Military Operational Medicine Research Program (MOMRP). This work was partially supported by the Office of Naval Research Global, Grant Number N62909-22-1-2008 (GS). Additionally, GS is supported by the Fonds de Recherche du Québec (Santé) Research Scholar Program.

REFERENCES

1. Ramar K, Malhotra RK, Carden KA, et al. Sleep is essential to health: an American Academy of Sleep Medicine position statement. J Clin Sleep Med 2021;17(10):2115–9.
2. Chattu VK, Manzar MD, Kumary S, et al. The global problem of insufficient sleep and its Serious public health Implications. Healthcare (Basel) 2018;7(1). https://doi.org/10.3390/healthcare7010001.
3. Stranges S, Tigbe W, Gomez-Olive FX, et al. Sleep problems: an emerging global epidemic? Findings from the INDEPTH WHO-SAGE study among more than 40,000 older adults from 8 countries across Africa and Asia. Sleep 2012; 35(8):1173–81.
4. Hafner M, Stepanek M, Taylor J, et al. Why Sleep Matters-The Economic Costs of Insufficient Sleep: A Cross-Country Comparative Analysis. Rand Health Q 2017;6(4):11.
5. Acquavella J, Mehra R, Bron M, et al. Prevalence of narcolepsy and other sleep disorders and frequency of diagnostic tests from 2013-2016 in insured patients actively seeking care. J Clin Sleep Med 2020;16(8):1255–63.
6. Cenat JM, Blais-Rochette C, Kokou-Kpolou CK, et al. Prevalence of symptoms of depression, anxiety, insomnia, posttraumatic stress disorder, and psychological distress among populations affected by the COVID-19 pandemic: a systematic review and meta-analysis. Psychiatry Res 2021;295: 113599.
7. Jahrami HA, Alhaj OA, Humood AM, et al. Sleep disturbances during the COVID-19 pandemic: a systematic review, meta-analysis, and meta-regression. Sleep Med Rev 2022;62:101591.
8. Marelli S, Castelnuovo A, Somma A, et al. Impact of COVID-19 lockdown on sleep quality in university students and administration staff. J Neurol 2021; 268(1):8–15.
9. Neculicioiu VS, Colosi IA, Costache C, et al. Time to sleep?-A review of the impact of the COVID-19 pandemic on sleep and mental health. Int J Environ Res Public Health 2022;(6):19. https://doi.org/10.3390/ijerph19063497.
10. Watson NF, Rosen IM, Chervin RD, et al. The Past is Prologue: the future of sleep medicine. J Clin Sleep Med 2017;13(1):127–35.
11. Shamim-Uzzaman QA, Bae CJ, Ehsan Z, et al. The use of telemedicine for the diagnosis and treatment of sleep disorders: an American Academy of Sleep Medicine update. J Clin Sleep Med 2021;17(5): 1103–7.

12. Aitken M. IQVIA Institute Report: Digital Health Trends 2021, July 22 2021. https://www.iqvia.com/insights/the-iqvia-institute/reports/digital-health-trends-2021.

13. Mobile Fact Sheet. Pew Research Center, 2022. https://www.pewresearch.org/internet/fact-sheet/mobile/. Accessed October 01, 2022.

14. Khosla S, Deak MC, Gault D, et al. Consumer sleep technology: an American Academy of sleep medicine position statement. J Clin Sleep Med 2018;14(5):877–80.

15. Ong AA, Gillespie MB. Overview of smartphone applications for sleep analysis. World J Otorhinolaryngol Head Neck Surg 2016;2(1):45–9.

16. Lorenz CP, Williams AJ. Sleep apps: what role do they play in clinical medicine? Curr Opin Pulm Med 2017;23(6):512–6.

17. Mansukhani MP, Kolla BP. Apps and fitness trackers that measure sleep: are they useful? Cleve Clin J Med 2017;84(6):451–6.

18. Guillodo E, Lemey C, Simonnet M, et al. Clinical applications of mobile health wearable-based sleep monitoring: systematic review. JMIR Mhealth Uhealth 2020;8(4):e10733.

19. Ananth S. Sleep apps: current limitations and challenges. Sleep Sci 2021;14(1):83–6.

20. Choi YK, Demiris G, Lin SY, et al. Smartphone applications to support sleep self-management: review and evaluation. J Clin Sleep Med 2018;14(10):1783–90.

21. Baron KG, Duffecy J, Berendsen MA, et al. Feeling validated yet? A scoping review of the use of consumer-targeted wearable and mobile technology to measure and improve sleep. Sleep Med Rev 2018;40:151–9.

22. Lee-Tobin PA, Ogeil RP, Savic M, et al. Rate my sleep: examining the information, function, and Basis in Empirical evidence within sleep applications for mobile devices. J Clin Sleep Med 2017;13(11):1349–54.

23. Baptista PM, Martin F, Ross H, et al. A systematic review of smartphone applications and devices for obstructive sleep apnea. Braz J Otorhinolaryngol 2022. https://doi.org/10.1016/j.bjorl.2022.01.004.

24. Stekl E, Klosterman G, Simonelli G, et al. 0095 Sleep enhancement technology in 2021: an Updated survey of apps. Sleep 2022;45(Supplement_1):A43.

25. Huberty J, Puzia ME, Larkey L, et al. Can a meditation app help my sleep? A cross-sectional survey of Calm users. PLoS One 2021;16(10):e0257518.

26. Huberty J, Puzia ME, Larkey L, et al. Use of the consumer-based meditation app Calm for sleep disturbances: cross-sectional survey study. JMIR Form Res 2020;4(11):e19508.

27. Huberty J, Green J, Glissmann C, et al. Efficacy of the mindfulness meditation mobile app "Calm" to reduce stress among College students: randomized controlled trial. JMIR Mhealth Uhealth 2019;7(6):e14273.

28. Bostock S, Crosswell AD, Prather AA, et al. Mindfulness on-the-go: effects of a mindfulness meditation app on work stress and well-being. J Occup Health Psychol 2019;24(1):127–38.

29. Zollars I, Poirier TI, Pailden J. Effects of mindfulness meditation on mindfulness, mental well-being, and perceived stress. Curr Pharm Teach Learn 2019;11(10):1022–8.

30. Rung AL, Oral E, Berghammer L, et al. Feasibility and Acceptability of a mobile mindfulness meditation intervention among Women: intervention study. JMIR Mhealth Uhealth 2020;8(6):e15943.

31. O'Daffer A, Colt SF, Wasil AR, et al. Efficacy and conflicts of interest in randomized controlled trials evaluating Headspace and Calm apps: systematic review. JMIR Ment Health 2022;9(9):e40924.

32. Chinoy ED, Cuellar JA, Huwa KE, et al. Performance of seven consumer sleep-tracking devices compared with polysomnography. Sleep 2021;(5):44.

33. Haghayegh S, Khoshnevis S, Smolensky MH, et al. Accuracy of Wristband Fitbit Models in assessing sleep: systematic review and meta-analysis. J Med Internet Res 2019;21(11):e16273.

34. Ding F, Cotton-Clay A, Fava L, et al. Polysomnographic validation of an under-mattress monitoring device in estimating sleep architecture and obstructive sleep apnea in adults. Sleep Med 2022;96:20–7

35. de Zambotti M, Rosas L, Colrain IM, et al. The sleep of the ring: Comparison of the OURA sleep tracker against polysomnography. Behav Sleep Med. Mar-Apr 2019;17(2):124–36.

36. Miller DJ, Sargent C, Roach GD. A validation of six wearable devices for estimating sleep, heart rate and heart rate Variability in healthy adults. Sensors 2022;(16):22.

37. Roberts DM, Schade MM, Mathew GM, et al. Detecting sleep using heart rate and motion data from multisensor consumer-grade wearables, relative to wrist actigraphy and polysomnography. Sleep 2020;43(7).

38. Edouard P, Campo D, Bartet P, et al. Validation of the Withings Sleep Analyzer, an under-the-mattress device for the detection of moderate-severe sleep apnea syndrome. J Clin Sleep Med 2021;17(6):1217–27.

39. Horger MN, Marsiliani R, DeMasi A, et al. Researcher Choices for infant sleep assessment: Parent report, actigraphy, and a Novel Video system. J Genet Psychol Jul-Aug 2021;182(4):218–35.

40. Patel P, Kim JY, Brooks LJ. Accuracy of a smartphone application in estimating sleep in children. Sleep Breath 2017;21(2):505–11.

41. Rusch HL, Rosario M, Levison LM, et al. The effect of mindfulness meditation on sleep quality: a

systematic review and meta-analysis of randomized controlled trials. Ann N Y Acad Sci 2019;1445(1): 5–16.

42. Feng F, Zhang Y, Hou J, et al. Can music improve sleep quality in adults with primary insomnia? A systematic review and network meta-analysis. Int J Nurs Stud 2018;77:189–96.

43. Alvarsson JJ, Wiens S, Nilsson ME. Stress recovery during exposure to nature sound and environmental noise. Int J Environ Res Public Health 2010;7(3): 1036–46.

44. Lee M, Song CB, Shin GH, et al. Possible effect of binaural beat combined with Autonomous sensory Meridian Response for Inducing sleep. Front Hum Neurosci 2019;13:425.

45. Durrani S, Cao S, Bo N, et al. A Feasibility study: testing whether a sleep application providing objective sleep data to physicians improves patient-physician Communication regarding sleep experiences, Habits, and behaviors. Adv Ther 2022;39(4):1612–29.

46. Stoyanov SR, Hides L, Kavanagh DJ, et al. Mobile app rating scale: a new tool for assessing the quality of health mobile apps. JMIR Mhealth Uhealth 2015; 3(1):e27.